NEUROLOGY - LABORATORY AND CLINICAL RESEARCH DEVELOPMENTS

RETT SYNDROME AND OTHER COMMUNICATION DISORDERS

SYMPTOMS, TREATMENT AND PROGNOSIS

NEUROLOGY - LABORATORY AND CLINICAL RESEARCH DEVELOPMENTS

Additional books in this series can be found on Nova's website under the Series tab.

Additional e-books in this series can be found on Nova's website under the e-book tab.

NEUROLOGY - LABORATORY AND CLINICAL RESEARCH DEVELOPMENTS

RETT SYNDROME AND OTHER COMMUNICATION DISORDERS

SYMPTOMS, TREATMENT AND PROGNOSIS

DANIEL L. KOLBY
EDITOR

New York

Library of Congress Cataloging-in-Publication Data

ISBN: 978-1-63463-920-0
Library of Congress Control Number: 2014960018

Published by Nova Science Publishers, Inc. † New York

Contents

Preface

This book discusses symptoms, treatment and prognosis of Rett Syndrome, as well as other related communication disorders.

Chapter 1 – Rett syndrome is a X-linked neurodevelopmental disorder that affects 1 in 10,000 females. It presents clinically with developmental regression at 6-18 months of age, with loss of acquired language and motor skills, leading to a complex lifelong syndrome characterised by intellectual disability; behavioural and neuropsychiatric disturbances; social withdrawal; hand stereotypies; epilepsy; autonomic dysfunction causing breathing irregularities and cardiac arrhythmias; muscle tone abnormalities leading to orthopaedic deformities such as scoliosis; and motor incoordination that causes gait disturbance and feeding difficulties which, along with a number of gastrointestinal problems, leads to growth failure and nutritional deficiencies.

Currently, the treatments for Rett syndrome are symptomatic and supportive. Given the complex functional consequences of the disease, this management plan requires an integrated multidisciplinary approach, incorporating medical management of the seizures, gastrointestinal dysfunction, spasticity and associated orthopaedic issues, breathing abnormalities, sleep disturbances and neuropsychiatric symptoms, as well as physical, occupational and speech and language therapy, nutritional supplementation and educational support, in order to generate a tailored programme that meets each child's individual needs and maximises her functional abilities.

However, since the discovery that over 90% of cases of Rett syndrome are caused by mutations of the X-linked *MECP2* gene, much has been learned about the basic biology underlying the disease. Methyl-CpG-binding protein 2 is a transcriptional regulator also involved in chromatin remodelling and RNA processing. Highly expressed in post-mitotic neurons, it is implicated in neuronal development and synaptic maturation. The discovery led to the development of *MECP2* knockout mouse models of Rett syndrome, which successfully recapitulate many features of the Rett syndrome phenotype, including delayed onset, motor dysfunction, cognitive impairment, breathing irregularities, EEG abnormalities and reduced lifespan. The subsequent discovery that this phenotype can be reversed by genetic restoration of *MECP2* function in mouse models suggests that the neuronal dysfunction that occurs in Rett syndrome is not permanent, and is amenable to treatment. This has led to a surge in research that seeks to identify therapies that reverse the disease process in mouse models and can subsequently be translated into therapies for human clinical trials.

These experimental therapeutic techniques include direct restoration of *MECP2* function by delivery of a replacement *MECP2* gene through gene therapy, by pharmacological reactivation of the silenced *MECP2* gene or by drug treatment that allows read-through of the mutated gene. Other strategies involve activation of signalling factors downstream from *MECP2*, most notably the neurotrophic factor BDNF. Finally, therapies are being developed that target the neurobiological consequences of *MECP2* dysfunction, by correcting the synaptic physiology and neurochemical systems altered in Rett syndrome, including the 5-HT, norepinephrine, acetylcholine, glutamate and GABA signalling systems.

Now, as the first wave of treatments first developed in Mecp2 mouse models reach the stage of clinical trial in human subjects, this review article reflects upon both the current and potential therapeutic strategies for treatment of Rett syndrome, by summarising the current management of Rett syndrome, describing therapies currently under clinical trial, and looking into the future at exciting new treatments being developed with the use of mouse models.

Chapter 2 – This chapter provides a literature overview concerning empirical studies aimed at promoting adaptive behaviors (e.g. communicative skills, locomotion) and reducing stereotypic behaviors (e.g. body rocking, hand clipping) in children with Rett syndrome and severe to profound developmental disabilities through rehabilitative programs based on cognitive-behavioral interventions and/or assistive technology, published in the last period (i.e. 2000-2014). A combined computerized and manual search was conducted to identify the empirical evidences that were retained for the overview. That is, 20 studies were selected for this purpose. Outcomes were largely positive and encouraging, although some failure occurred. A second goal of the chapter was to point out strengths and weakness of the aforementioned studies. Finally, a third objective was to emphasize critical issues and future questions to be addressed for the future research and practice in this topic area. Clinical, educational and psychological implications of the findings are also discussed.

Chapter 3 – In 1990 Dieler R. et al., described in conjunctival, muscle and peripheral artery biopsies examined by light and electron microscopy, amorphous and membranous electron-dense deposits in capillaries of Rett syndrome (RTT) patients. Subclinical myocardial dysfunctions in RTT have been recently described in the patients, together with modification of the perfusion index. The presence of cold hands and feet, and blue, is a non-neurological phenotype that characterize RTT up to now not well explained. In order to evaluate the state of the microvascularity in RTT the authors have performed a complexity analysis of the microvasculature in the patients. By nailfold videocapillaroscopy they observed dilated capillaries and irregular, chaotic microvascular patterns.

To quantify these features The authors have performed a nonlinear analysis of the images. Entropy resulted higher in Rett females than in sex- and age-matched healthy individuals ($p<0.001$). In RTT patients subtle modifications of the microvascular system are present, aspects that deserve to be deeply investigated.

In: Rett Syndrome and Other Communication ... ISBN: 978-1-63463-920-0
Editor: Daniel L. Kolby

Chapter 1

Treating Rett Syndrome: Current Approaches and New Treatments

***D. Tropea*[1], *S. Wrigley*[2] *and G. Pini*[3*]**
[1]Neuropsychiatric Genetics, Trinity Centre for Health Sciences, St James Hospital, Dublin, Ireland
[2]Medical School, Trinity College Dublin, College Green, D2, Dublin, Ireland
[3]Tuscany Rett Centre, Versilia Hospital, Lido di Camaiore (LU), Italy

Abstract

Rett syndrome is a X-linked neurodevelopmental disorder that affects 1 in 10,000 females. It presents clinically with developmental regression at 6-18 months of age, with loss of acquired language and motor skills, leading to a complex lifelong syndrome characterised by intellectual disability; behavioural and neuropsychiatric disturbances; social withdrawal; hand stereotypies; epilepsy; autonomic dysfunction causing breathing irregularities and cardiac arrhythmias; muscle tone

* Corresponding Author: Dr. Giorgio Pini, Tuscany Rett Centre, Versilia Hospital, Lido di Camaiore (LU), Italy, Phone: +39 0584 6059552, Fax: +39 0584 6059801, Email: g.pini@usl12.toscana.it.

abnormalities leading to orthopaedic deformities such as scoliosis; and motor incoordination that causes gait disturbance and feeding difficulties which, along with a number of gastrointestinal problems, leads to growth failure and nutritional deficiencies.

Currently, the treatments for Rett syndrome are symptomatic and supportive. Given the complex functional consequences of the disease, this management plan requires an integrated multidisciplinary approach, incorporating medical management of the seizures, gastrointestinal dysfunction, spasticity and associated orthopaedic issues, breathing abnormalities, sleep disturbances and neuropsychiatric symptoms, as well as physical, occupational and speech and language therapy, nutritional supplementation and educational support, in order to generate a tailored programme that meets each child's individual needs and maximises her functional abilities.

However, since the discovery that over 90% of cases of Rett syndrome are caused by mutations of the X-linked *MECP2* gene, much has been learned about the basic biology underlying the disease. Methyl-CpG-binding protein 2 is a transcriptional regulator also involved in chromatin remodelling and RNA processing. Highly expressed in post-mitotic neurons, it is implicated in neuronal development and synaptic maturation. The discovery led to the development of *MECP2* knockout mouse models of Rett syndrome, which successfully recapitulate many features of the Rett syndrome phenotype, including delayed onset, motor dysfunction, cognitive impairment, breathing irregularities, EEG abnormalities and reduced lifespan. The subsequent discovery that this phenotype can be reversed by genetic restoration of *MECP2* function in mouse models suggests that the neuronal dysfunction that occurs in Rett syndrome is not permanent, and is amenable to treatment. This has led to a surge in research that seeks to identify therapies that reverse the disease process in mouse models and can subsequently be translated into therapies for human clinical trials.

These experimental therapeutic techniques include direct restoration of *MECP2* function by delivery of a replacement *MECP2* gene through gene therapy, by pharmacological reactivation of the silenced *MECP2* gene or by drug treatment that allows read-through of the mutated gene. Other strategies involve activation of signalling factors downstream from *MECP2*, most notably the neurotrophic factor BDNF. Finally, therapies are being developed that target the neurobiological consequences of *MECP2* dysfunction, by correcting the synaptic physiology and neurochemical systems altered in Rett syndrome, including the 5-HT, norepinephrine, acetylcholine, glutamate and GABA signalling systems.

Now, as the first wave of treatments first developed in Mecp2 mouse models reach the stage of clinical trial in human subjects, this review article reflects upon both the current and potential therapeutic strategies for treatment of Rett syndrome, by summarising the current management of Rett syndrome, describing therapies currently under clinical trial, and looking into the future at exciting new treatments being developed with the use of mouse models.

Introduction

Rett syndrome is a X-linked neurodevelopmental disorder that develops in girls during early childhood. These girls show normal developmental progress during the first 6-18 months of life, acquiring gross motor skills such as walking, fine motor skills, and basic language and communication skills, while also showing normal social skills including smiling responsively.

However, over time they demonstrate developmental stagnation (Stage 1) followed by regression (Stage 2), with loss of acquired skills (Hagberg et al., 1986). The earliest sign is deceleration is head growth, leading to microcephaly by the second year of life (Weaving et al., 2005). This is accompanied by weight loss and failure to thrive, in the absence of poor feeding or malabsorption. The girls develop generalised muscle hypotonia, leading to abnormalities in posture, and loss of motor coordination, causing ataxia and gait disturbance. Notably, they lose purposeful use of their hands, and develop characteristic hand stereotypies, including hand-washing, wringing, clapping and tapping. There is evident loss of language, and social withdrawal, with development of autistic features such as lack of eye contact and unresponsiveness to social cues. While Stage 2 is characterised by rapid cognitive and motor regression, Stage 3 describes a period of partial recovery. There is typically some improvement in social interaction and acquisition of some basic skills (Ellaway et al., 2001). Stage 3, beginning during the 4th year of life, is also characterised by development of autonomic dysfunction. This includes breathing abnormalities such as tachypnoea, hyperventilation, breath-holding, apnoea, Valsava manoeuvres, and aerophagia with abdominal bloating. These breathing dysrhythmias are thought to reflect developmental immaturity of the brainstem. They become evident towards the end of the period of developmental regression (Stage 2). Other features of autonomic dysfunction include small cold, blue hands and feet, oropharyngeal dysfunction, and cardiac arrhythmias such as prolonged QT intervals (Chahrour et al., 2007). There is normal sympathetic function, but reduced parasympathetic function remains at neonatal levels throughout life. Another important feature of Rett syndrome at this stage is the occurrence of seizures, which ranges in severity from easily-controlled to intractable epilepsy

(Chahrour et al., 2007). It is often a prominent management issue during childhood and adolescence, decreasing in severity thereafter. In general, Stage 4, which describes the stabilisation of cognitive function, is reached by 10 years of age. The problems associated with breathing abnormalities and seizures become less prominent, and the mild cognitive improvement that occurs in Stage 3 reaches a plateau (Ellaway et al., 2001). There is continued motor deterioration, with progressive replacement of muscle hypotonia by generalised rigidity, spasticity, and dystonia. This leads to a number of orthopaedic problems, such as the development of joint contractures and postural deformities, with worsening of scoliosis. This interferes with mobility and ambulation, which has implications for bone health mineralisation (Motil et al., 2008). While these hyperkinetic movement disorders characterise the clinical picture early in life, bradykinesia and other parkinsonian features develop later in life (Fitzgerald et al., 1990). Other management problems include sleep disturbance, agitation, anxiety, low-mood and self-injurious behaviour. There is also gastrointestinal dysfunction including gastroesophageal reflux and constipation, as well as problems with feeding, leading to growth failure and nutritional deficiencies including osteopenia.

Over 95% cases of typical Rett Syndrome are caused by mutations of the X-linked methyl-CpG-binding protein 2 (MeCP2) (Chapleau et al., 2013). A small proportion of cases are caused by mutation of the *CDLK5* gene, which is associated with earlier onset of seizure disorder (Weaving et al., 2005). However, given that the vast majority of cases are caused by *MECP2* mutations, and research into treatment development is largely based on the *MECP2* mutant model, it is this genetic form of Rett syndrome that will be discussed here. The Mecp2 protein is widely expressed in many cell types, and is particularly abundant in neurons. It is a transcriptional repressor, and is involved in CNS development, though its exact role remains unclear. Genetic restoration of MeCP2 (Guy et al., 2007; Giacometti et al., 2007) or activation of downstream signalling proteins (Chang et al., 2006; Tropea et al., 2009) has been shown to rescue the phenotype in mouse models of Rett syndrome. However, the pathological mechanisms underlying Rett syndrome are only just being elucidated. Therefore, current treatment strategies are supportive, targeting the symptoms rather than the disease. Given the wide range of clinical issues that arise in Rett syndrome, symptomatic treatment requires an integrated multidisciplinary approach, incorporating physiotherapy, occupational therapy and speech and language therapy, with input from specialist nurses, dieticians, paediatricians, neurologists, orthopaedic surgeons and psychiatrists, with an emphasis on psychosocial support for families, and on the development of a structured educational plan for the girls, tailored to support their specific needs and maximise their individual skills and abilities. However, the degree of practical support offered to children with Rett syndrome varies from country to country, and while these measures are important in improving quality of life, they do not alter the course of the underlying disease. A review of the current treatment strategies for management of the different clinical issues commonly seen in Rett syndrome is given in the following paragraphs and summarized in Table 1.

Symptomatic Management

Breathing Irregularities

A prominent feature of Rett syndrome is breathing dysfunction, including hyperventilation, deep breathing, rapid shallow breathing, apnoea, aerophagia with abdominal bloating, breath-holding and Valsava maneuver. Other features of autonomic dysfunction include heart rate dysregulation during wakefulness (Weese-Mayer et al., 2006), due to low cardiac vagal tone, similar to neonatal levels, and low baroreceptor reflex sensitivity, leading to unopposed sympathetic activity on blood pressure and heart rate (Kerr et al., 1999; Julu et al., 2001). The reduced parasympathetic activity seen in Rett syndrome leads to excessive swings in blood pressure and heart rate during episodes of hyperventilation, Valsalva breathing or inadequate breathing (Kerr et al., 1999; Julu et al., 2001). These episodes therefore carry a risk of sudden death due to cardiac arrhythmias or arrest (Julu et al., 2001). These respiratory abnormalities may cause up to 26% deaths in Rett syndrome (Julu et al., 1997; Kerr et al., 1997).Therefore, adequate management of breathing abnormalities form an important part of the treatment plan for patients with Rett syndrome.

These breathing dysrhythmias, along with reduced vagal tone with resultant sympatho-parasympathetic disproportion and poor autonomic integration, are thought to reflect developmental immaturity of the brainstem (Julu et al., 2001). This periodic breathing develops in girls aged 3-5 years, and is most problematic between the age of 5 and 15 years (Percy, 2014). It can interfere with feeding, and can lead to episodes that mimic seizure events. The type of breathing abnormalities that occur appear to be age-related, with forceful breathing and apneusis usually occurring in children under 5 years, rapid shallow breathing occurring in girls aged under 18, and Valsava breathing occurring in young adults (Julu et al., 2001).

In Rett syndrome, three types of breathers have been identified; forceful breathers, feeble breathers and apneustic breathers, all of whom could develop Valsava breathing (Julu et al., 2008). Forceful breathers develop chronic respiratory alkalosis, due to low levels of CO_2. Episodes of forceful breathing can be interrupted by use of a re-breather bag to increase CO_2 levels. Long-term management of the respiratory alkalosis involves use of Carbogen (5% CO_2 in oxygen) (Julu et al., 2008). On the other hand, feeble breathers develop chronic respiratory acidosis due to increased blood CO_2 levels. Stimulation of breathing is achieved by treatment with oral theophylline (Julu et al., 2008). The apneusis seen in Rett syndrome is thought to result from dysfunction of seritonergic neurons in the brainstem, as termination of respiration depends on activation of 5-HT1A receptors (Kerr et al., 1999). Therefore, apenustic breathers respond to oral buspirone, a 5-HT1A agonist. BiPAP may also be considered in these patients to control the tidal volume, though clinical experience is limited (Julu et al., 2008). All these breathing phenotypes may by complicated by Valsava manoeuvres, characterised by swinging changes in heart rate and blood pressure, episodes of which can be confused with seizures. Correct diagnosis of these episodes is essential in order to avoid unnecessary anticonvulsant therapy (Julu et al., 2008). These approaches to arresting and modifying the periodic breathing show limited success. Newer clinical trials and experimental molecular therapeutic methods are summarised further on in this review.

Abnormalties in Muscle Tone: Pharmacological Management

In Rett syndrome, muscle tone is reduced during infancy and early childhood. This develops into hypertonia, with generalised rigidity, spasticity and dystonic posturing. These motor abnormalities cause significant functional impairment and associated orthopaedic problems such as chronic pain, reduced mobility, neurogenic deformities, joint instability and fixed contractures, as well as skin breakdown in those who are non-ambulatory. Additionally, oropharyngeal dystonia (bruxism) contributes to impaired feeding and failure to thrive, while reduced mobility contributes to osteopenia. Therefore, treatment of spasticity is essential in attempts to maximise the functional abilities of girls with Rett syndrome.

Treatments for spasticity in children have been most widely studied in relation to cerebral palsy. Oral antispasmodic medications include benzodiazepines, baclofen, dantrolene sodium and the $\alpha 2$ agonists, tinzanidine and clonidine. Low-dose benzodiazepines such as diazepam or clozapam are effective in the treatment of spasticity in the paediatric population (Krach et al., 2001; Dahlin et al., 1993). However, in the long term, benzodiazepine treatment poses a risk of dependence and tolerance, and also causes side-effects including sedation and weakness which limit the clinician's ability to increase the dose and allow maximal control of spasticity (Krach et al., 2001; Chung et al., 2011). While benzodiazepines are centrally-acting agents that potentiate GABAa receptors, dantrolene acts peripherally on skeletal muscle, and may therefore be used in combination with benzodiazepines. It has been shown to be effective in reducing spasticity in children with cerebral palsy (Badell, 1991). Dosing of dantrolene is also limited due to its risk of serious adverse events including hepatotoxicity (Krach et al., 2001; Chung et al., 2011). Tizanidine and clonidine are centrally-acting α2 adrenergic agonists which are used as short-acting muscle relaxants. Tizanidine is safe for use in paediatric populations (Hennessy et al., 2009), and is as effective as diazepam and baclofen in tone reduction (Krach et al., 2001). It is shown to be effective in combination with botulinum toxin A injections (Dai et al., 2008). Clonidine has also been shown to be an effective antispasmodic agent in combination with baclofen (Donovan et al., 1988). However, their side-effects and the need for frequent dosing are limiting factors to its use (Chung et al., 2011). Finally, baclofen is a GABAb agonist that is one of the most commonly used antispasmodic medications in children (Lubshc et al., 2006). Its efficacy has been proven in children with cerebral palsy (Milla et al., 1977; Scheinberg et al., 2006). However, its use is limited because of its systemic side-effects including weakness, sedation, behavioural changes and ataxia (Dan et al., 2010). Its adverse effects may be avoided by administration by intrathecal injections into the subarachnoid space (Mathur et al., 2014). It is effective in the treatment of spasticity of cerebral origin, particularly lower limb spasticity (Armstrong et al., 1997), and shows proven efficacy in children (Hoving et al., 2009). It is suitable for long-term use (Albright et al., 2003; Mathur et al., 2014). It allows for functional improvement and is cost-effective (Sampson et al., 2002), with minimal long-term side-effects. The adverse events that occur are mainly linked to pump placement and include infections and CSF leaks (Motta et al., 2014). Additionally, it reduces the need for subsequent orthopaedic surgery (Gertszten et al., 1998). In particular, the intrathecal baclofen pump has been shown to be an appropriate option in the treatment of severe spasticity associated with Rett syndrome (Kadyan et al., 2003). Thus, intrathecal baclofen should be considered for patients who fail to respond to physical therapy and oral medication (Dan et al., 2010). Another treatment option for management of spasticity is injection of botulinum toxin A, which causes localised long-lasting muscle paralysis, inhibiting muscle spasm and causing pain relief. Botulinum toxin injection into the gastrocnemius muscle has been shown to reduce lower limb spasticity and allow for functional improvement in walking in children with cerebral palsy (Koman et al., 2000; Simpson et al., 2008; Molenaers et al., 2013). It is also effective for the treatment of equinus deformity (Simpson et al., 2008). Upper limb botulinum treatment is also associated with reduced spasticity, increased range of movement and functional improvement (Simpson et al., 2008; Lee et al., 2013).

Abnormalities in Tone: Non-Pharmacological Management

The muscular imbalance that occurs in Rett syndrome and other disorders characterised by spasticity leads to muscle contracture. As the child grows, these muscle contractures lead to bony deformities. Therefore, while the pharmacotherapy described above aids the treatment of spasticity, long-term management also requires a combination of physiotherapy, serial casting, orthoses and finally surgical intervention. Physiotherapy encourages stretching of muscles, strengthening them and preserving range of movement (Larrson et al., 2001). Similarly, serial casting promotes stretching of muscles, which is a stimulus for muscle growth (Woo, 2001). This prevents the development of contractures.

Additionally, orthotic devices are useful in maintaining neutral positions of distal extremities, thereby preventing the development of postural deformities (Percy, 2014). In particular, ankle-foot orthoses are used to improve gait in children with spasticity disorders. Ankle-foot orthoses prevent excessive plantar flexion resulting from increased lower limb spasticity, thereby stabilising the joints of the hindfoot, and preventing foot deformities and joint contractures by maintaining foot alignment (Woo, 2001).

These management options may be combined with the oral or injectable drug treatments described above to relieve spasticity and allow normal stretching and weight-bearing, which facilitates normal muscle development, thereby delaying or preventing surgical intervention. For instance, the efficacy of ankle-foot orthoses described above can be enhanced by botulinum injections into the gastrocnemius muscle to prevent equinus foot deformities (Sees et al., 2013). Once physiotherapy, bracing, oral antispasmodics and nerve blocks are no longer effective, surgical interventions are required for spasticity-induced deformities.

Surgical interventions include tendon lengthening, tendon transfer, bony osteotomy and normalising rotation with fusion of joints (Woo et al., 2001) (Lynn et al., 2009). Tendon lengthening increases passive range of movement. Strengthening of antagonist muscle groups by tendon transfer corrects the muscular imbalance that leads to postural deformities. When muscle imbalance leads to deformity, bony osteotomy is indicated to restore normal bony architecture. Specific deformities that most commonly result from spasticity include lower-limb rotational deformities, presenting as in-toeing or out-toeing, hip dysplasia and equionovalgus foot deformities, all of which are surgically managed by a combination of tendon lengthening, tendon transfer and osteotomy (Woo et al., 2001) If osteotomy is not possible, and the deformity cannot be braced, joint fusion to stabilise the joint of performed (Woo et al., 2001).

In Rett syndrome, the abnormalities in tone, posture and locomotion leading to loss of gross motor function not only cause the malpositions, joint contractures and foot deformities described above, but also lead to scoliosis and loss of ambulation (Larrson et al., 2001) (Hanks, 1990), the management of which are described below.

Scoliosis

Scoliosis is a common complication of Rett syndrome. Scoliosis is present in 8% of children aged less than 5 years, and over 80% girls aged over 16 years. One study showed that the mean age of onset was 9.8 years, with 75% patients developing scoliosis by 13 years (Ager et al., 2006). Factors that predict onset of scoliosis include impaired development before 6 months, reduced mobility at 10 months, and a history of having never walked. Scoliosis in Rett syndrome is neurogenic (Lidstrom et al., 1994), resulting from the hypotonia, generalised weakness and muscular insufficiency that manifests in Rett syndrome. Compared with the idiopathic form of scoliosis, it shows earlier onset and more rapid progression that does not necessarily halt with cessation of growth (Ager et al., 2006).

Close observation is required to monitor the progression of the scoliosis with 6 monthly Xrays to measure the curvature (Cobb's angle) of the spine. Bracing is advised when the curvature exceeds 25° (Hagberg et al., 1993) (Percy, 2014), to slow the progression of scoliosis during puberty. However, given that the scoliosis in Rett syndrome is neurogenic in origin, and therefore shows more rapid progression, bracing may be considered at an even earlier stage. Typically, the braces are worn for 23 hours per day until growth cessation. However, given that curve progression usually continues beyond growth cessation in Rett syndrome, surgery is often necessary. Surgery is strongly recommended when the curvature exceeds 40° (Hagberg et al., 1993; Percy, 2014). Surgical options include anterior/posterior spinal fusion surgery, posterior instrumentation without fusion, or vertebral expanding prosthetic titanium rib.

Surgical instrumentation shows a definite improvement in quality of life, though one study reports improvements in posture and feeding, but not ambulation (Kerr et al., 2003).

Ambulation

80% of girls with Rett syndrome acquire the ability to walk, but 30% of these will lose the ability during the period of developmental regression, so that, overall, about 50% of girls with Rett syndrome remain ambulatory (Percy, 2014). Ambulation is important for bone density mineralisation and development of muscle strength and correct posture. Therefore, for those who do not walk, weight-bearing exercises are recommended, with the use of standing frames or gait-trainers (Lotan et al., 2004; Percy, 2014).

Behavioural Disturbances

This is a common management problem in children with Rett syndrome. One study conducted a survey to assess the extent of emotional and behavioural problems in Rett syndrome, and reported that 76% patients had episodes of anxiety, 70% suffered from low mood, and 49% demonstrated self-injurious behaviour (Sansom et al., 1993).

The selective serotonin reuptake inhibitors (SSRIs) are the most widely used and successful agents in the management of anxiety and mood disorders (Namerow et al., 2003; Chapleau et al., 2013). They are first-line for treatment of anxiety or mood disorder in children, including children with pervasive developmental disorders (Emslie et al., 2002; Namerow et al., 2003).

They are also used to treat the core features of autism spectrum disorder including social withdrawal, restricted interests and repetitive behaviours.

However, a Cochrane review reports that there is currently no evidence for their use here (Williams et al., 2013). Antidepressants such as clomipramine, sertraline, fluvoxamine and citalopram are used in the treatment of obsessive-compulsive disorder in adults, and therefore the treatment of repetitive behaviours in Autism Spectrum Disorders (ASDs) largely rests on the use of these SSRIs (Hampson et al., 2012). However, there is insufficient evidence to support their use in the treatment of repetitive behaviours in children with ASDs (King et al., 2009).

Risperidone is useful both in the treatment of self-injurious behaviour and behavioural disturbances (Percy, 2014) (Shea et al., 2004). Aripiprazole is another antipsychotic that was shown to be effective and well-tolerated (Marcus et al., 2009) (Owen et al., 2009). Clinical trials also demonstrate that parental training in additional to risperidone/aripiprazole therapy was superior to risperidone therapy alone in managing behavioural problems in children with Rett syndrome (Aman et al., 2009). These are currently the only drugs approved to treat irritability in ASD (Hampson et al., 2012).

Non-pharmacological therapies are also employed in the management of hand stereotypies, agitation and self-injurious behaviour. While behavioural techniques are ineffective in reducing stereotypic hand movements in girls with Rett syndrome (Naganuma et al., 1998), hand and elbow splints are used to restrict purposeless, stereotypic hand movements, and to prevent self-injurous behaviour. A study of their use in eight children showed that they improved socialisation (Aron et al., 1990). Splinting of the hands prevents them from acting as a source of distraction, allowing these girls to better interact with their environment. One study reports reduced stereotypic hand movements and improved interaction with toys with the use of elbow orthoses, and no change with the use of hand splints (Sharpe et al., 1992).

Seizures

Seizures are common in Rett syndrome. They rarely occur before the age of 2 years, and EEG recordings during infancy are normal. Seizures typically become prominent during Stage 3 of the disease, between the ages of 2 and 10 years (Chahrour et al., 2007). Epilepsy in Rett syndrome is associated with increased clinical severity of the disease, with patients showing greater impairment of hand use, communication and ambulation (Glaze et al., 2010). The electroencephalogram readings in a patient with Rett syndrome are always abnormal after 2 years of age, showing a slowing in background activity, a decrease or loss of posterior dominant rhythm, and recurrent spike and slow wave activity (Percy, 2002). However, it is important that EEG changes are only treated if there is a clinical correlate because, despite these epileptiform changes on EEG, not all patients develop clinical manifestations of epilepsy. In fact, seizure events are overestimated in Rett syndrome, as a number of behavioural patterns and episodes of autonomic dysregulation or "brainstem events" mimic seizures. In one study, 23 out of 55 caretakers identified non-seizure activities such as twitching, jerking, head turning, staring, laughing, pupillary dilation, breath-holding and hyperventilation as seizure events (Glaze et al., 1998). Conversely, out of 13 patients who had clinical seizure events during the study, only in 5 patients were the events recognised by caretakers. Misdiagnosis of seizures can lead to inappropriate anti-convulsant therapy. Therefore, careful diagnosis of seizures is recommended. The only way to differentiate between seizures and brainstem events is to perform simultaneous neurophysiological studies of both brainstem and cortical activity during these events by video-EEG monitoring (Julu et al., 2001) (Julu et al., 2008).

While correct diagnosis of seizures in Rett syndrome is problematic, seizure control is usually not difficult. The most commonly used drugs used singly or in combination are valproate, carbamazepine and lamotrigine (Percy, 2002; Jian et al., 2007; Chapleau et al., 2013), which are first-line for treatment of seizures in the paediatric population. Sulthiame has also been shown to be effective (Huppke et al., 2007). Other drugs used include oxcarbazepine, levetiracetam, topiramate and clozabam (Percy, 2014) (Nissencorn et al., 2010). Overall, drug-resistant epilepsy occurs in 38% cases of epilepsy in Rett syndrome (Pintaudi et al., 2010). For these cases, alternative therapies such as vagal nerve stimulation and ketogenic diets are under investigation, and have shown efficacy in many cases ((Keane et al., 2006; Wilfong et al., 2006; Neal et al., 2008; Dressler et al., 2010; Percy, 2014).

Sleep Disturbance

Disturbance of sleep patterns is a common feature of Rett syndrome. It typically develops during stage III of the disorder (McArthur et al., 1998). It includes irregular sleep times, sleep-onset latency, periodic night-time awakening with disruptive behaviour, and reduced total sleep time. While sleep disorders affect 10-30% of all children, they affect 80% of children with Rett syndrome (McArthur et al., 1998).

There is increasing evidence that sleep disturbances in children with autism spectrum disorders are linked to defects in melatonin secretion (Gionnotti et al., 2006). Studies show that melatonin causes a significant reduction in sleep-latency in children with neurodevelopmental disorders, including Rett syndrome (Miyamoto et al., 1999; Phillips et al., 2004; Gionnotti et al., 2006). Melatonin treatment is well-tolerated, with no significant adverse effects (Phillips et al., 2004). In all, melatonin is the safest and most widely validated treatment of sleep disorder in children with neurodevelopmental disabilities (Holloway et al., 2011). Another alternative is ramelton, a potent M1/M2 melatonin receptor agonist. It is a well-tolerated and effective drug for treatment of insomnia in adults (Erman et al., 2006; Roth et al., 2006; Zammitt et al., 2007; Wang-Weigand et al., 2009), though its use in children has not been widely assessed.

Other commonly prescribed drugs for treatment of sleep disturbance in neurodevelopmental disorders are antihistamines, α-adrenoreceptor agonists, chloral hydrate, antidepressants, antipsychotics, benzodiazepines, and non-benzodiazepine drugs (zolpidem, zopiclone) (Holloway et al., 2011).

Antihistamines used in the treatment of sleep disturbance include diphenhydramine, trimeprazine and niaprazine. While results for diphenhydramine were mixed (Russo et al., 1976; Paul et al., 2004; Merenstein et al., 2006), studies show that trimeprazine and niaprazine are effective for sleep disturbance in children (Siminoff et al., 1987; France et al., 1991; Ottaviano et al., 1991). Only niaprazine has been studied for use in children with developmental disorders and was shown to be effective (Rossi et al., 1999).

Clonidine is a centrally-acting presynaptic α adrenoreceptor used clinically as an antihypertensive. It is also used in children for the treatment of ADHD, and has shown to effectively treat insomnia in children in retrospective case review studies (Ingrassia et al., 2005; Ming et al., 2008). However, studies in adults showed that it caused a reduction in REM sleep. This may impact on memory consolidation and skill development.

While benzodiazepines are known to be effective hypnotics, they are not recommended for use in children because of their adverse side-effects (Holloway et al., 2011). The non-benzodiazepine "Z drugs" (zolpidem and zolpiclone) have less potential for abuse and dependence. Results for use of zolpidem in children have been mixed, with studies showing no changes or only small improvements in sleep-onset latency (Armour et al., 2008; Blumer et al., 2009).

The use of a number of antidepressants in the treatment of insomnia has also been assessed. Trazodone is a serotonin antagonist reuptake inhibitor with antidepressant and sedative properties commonly prescribed in children with developmental disorders (Holloway et al., 2011), though no randomised controlled trials have been performed. In an open-label study, trazodone was shown to improve sleep in young children with opsoclonus-myoclonus disorder (Pranzatelli et al., 2005). Mirtazepine is a presynaptic α adrenoreceptor blocker that increases levels of noradrenaline. It is known to have sedative properties, and in one open-label study it caused improvement in sleep parameters in 31% children (Posey et al., 2001). In adults, it improves sleep maintenance and prolongs slow-wave sleep.

Tricyclic antidepressants such as imipramine and amitryptilene are used in the treatment of insomnia, but are not recommended, as imipramine causes increased alertness and amitryptilene causes a reduction in REM sleep (Holloway et al., 2011). These medications should be avoided in Rett syndrome because they cause prolongation of the QT interval. Risperidone is used in the treatment of self-injurious behaviour in Rett syndrome, and has also been assessed in the treatment of sleep disturbance, with some positive results. Other antipsychotics are not recommended (Holloway et al., 2011). Finally, chloral hydrate, while considered an effective sedative, is often unsuitable for children due to its strong taste (Percy, 2014).

More studies are required to examine the efficacy of medications used for sleep disturbance in Rett syndrome, with greater emphasis on examining the effect of these medications on sleep architecture, as reductions in REM and slow-wave sleep could affect memory consolidation and skill acquisition, which is already impaired in children with Rett syndrome. In general, melatonin, antihistamines and clonidine appear to be the most widely prescribed medications, while newer medications such as trazodone and mirtazapine appear promising but require further characterisation.

Gastrointestinal Problems

There is abnormal functioning of the digestive system in 74% cases of Rett syndrome, including gastroesophageal reflux, constipation, failure to thrive and malnutrition (Lotan et al., 2006). Along with other factors that interfere with feeding, this contributes to the pervasive growth failure and nutritional deficiencies that occur in Rett syndrome.

Gastroesophageal reflux disease (GORD) is extremely common in Rett syndrome. It can cause oesophagitis, oesophageal strictures and lung aspiration, and can also cause unexplained irritability and distress that the child is unable to communicate, contributing to the behavioural disturbances that occur in Rett syndrome. Upright positioning during feeds, and thickening of feeds, is the initial treatment for gastroesophageal reflux. However, thickening of feed appears to reduce the volume but not the frequency of reflux episodes (Yvan et al., 2009). Best practice guidelines for treatment of gastroesophageal reflux in children indicate that acid-suppressant therapy is the mainstay of treatment. This includes proton pump inhibitors (PPIs), such as lanzoprazole, and histamine receptor 2 antagonists, such as cimetidine. PPIs are superior to HR2As (Yvan et al., 2009), given that HR2As demonstrate reduced efficacy following long-term use. However, efficacy of PPIs in treatment of GOR in infants aged under 1 year has not been proven. Antacids may be used for short-term symptomatic relief but are not recommended for long-term use. Surgical management by fundoplication is recommended in cases where GORD is refractory to medical therapy or where there is a high risk of aspiration.

Hypoactive bowel function, including delayed gastric emptying and constipation, is another feature of gatointestinal dysfunction in Rett syndrome. Delayed gastric emptying which is best managed by prokinetic agents including erythromycin or bethanecol (Percy, 2014). Prokinetic agents such as metocloperamide and domperidone should be avoided, as their dopamine-blocking actions could precipitate or worsen movement disorders in girls with Rett syndrome (Percy, 2014).

Constipation affects all girls with Rett syndrome. It results from both the poor bowel function relating to the disorder, and from a number of contributing factors such as reduced physical activity, reduced fluid intake, diet and medication (Lotan et al., 2006). Treatment of constipation involves disimpacting the bowel followed by maintenance of a regular bowel movement routine. Currently, there is insufficient evidence to recommend one method of bowel disimpaction over another (Felt et al., 1999), and various strategies may be employed, including the use of enemas (mineral oil, hypertonic phosphate, saline), or oral medications such as polyethylene glycol electrolyte solution, high-dose mineral oil, osmotic laxatives (e.g. lactulose, sorbitol) or stimulant laxatives (bisacodyl, senna) (Felt et al., 1999) (Baker et al., 1999). Maintenance therapy consists of dietary intervention, behavioural modifications, and short-term laxative use to establish regular bowel movements. Dietary interventions include increased fluid intake and implementation of a high-fibre diet. Behavioural modifications involve increased physical activity where possible, and regular toileting, with the goal that the child sit on the toilet for 5-10 minutes at least 3-4 times per day, usually after meals and at bed-time, recorded with use of a defecation chart. Medication during the maintenance phase is highly beneficial. Recommended laxatives include lubricants such as mineral oil, or osmotic laxatives such as lactulose (Felt et al., 1999). Stimulant laxatives, used for bowel disimpaction, are not recommended for the maintenance phase. The use of laxative medications should be restricted as dependence can develop. However, months of treatment may be necessary before medication can be weaned (Loton et al., 2006). There is now an increasing awareness of gallbladder disease in patients with Rett syndrome (Percy et al., 2005), and includes gallbladder dysfunction and gallstones. The frequency of gallbladder dysfunction is girls with Rett syndrome is approximately 3% (Motil et al., 2012). It represents another cause of unexplained pain and irritability in affected girls. Cholcystectomy is indicated when gallstones are identified, or when gallbladder dysfunction leads to an ejection fraction less than 35-40% (Percy, 2014).

Feeding, Nutrition and Growth

Growth failure is a prominent feature of Rett syndrome. The first sign is head growth deceleration, which begins as early as 1 month of age, leading to an occipito-frontal circumference approaching the 2nd centile by 2 years of age (Tarquino et al., 2012) (Schultz et al., 1993). Weight gain slows, falling below the average for a normal population, by 6 months of age, so that by 12-13 years the median weight is below the 2nd centile. Height or length deceleration occurs by 17 months of age (Tarquino et al., 2012), so that median height is below the 2nd centile by 12 years of age. There are similar declines in hand and foot growth, though the feet are more affected (Schultz et al., 1988).

Lower metabolic rates may account for the growth deficits seen in girls with Rett syndrome (Motil et al., 1994). However, failure to thrive and ongoing growth impairment in Rett syndrome is also linked to feeding difficulties, as this leads to a mean energy intake that is only 66.9% that of the US recommendations for age (Thommessen et al., 2008). The gastrointestinal and feeding difficulties observed in this population results from a number of factors and therefore require a multidisciplinary assessment. Breathing abnormalities, such as apnoea and hyperventilation interfere with feeding, while aerophagia leads to abdominal bloating. Oropharyngeal dysfunction, such as immature chewing patterns and dysphagia also cause impaired feeding and increase the risk of aspiration. Gastrointestinal problems such as GOR, delayed gastric emptying and constipation interfere with feeding by prolonging mealtimes, and causing pain, leading to refusal to feed. Gastrointestinal and feeding problems are further exacerbated by postural misalignment and muscle tone abnormalities. While each of these issues needs to be addressed in order to facilitate effective feeding, additional strategies are employed to prevent nutritional deficiencies and promote growth. Early involvement of a speech and language therapist may help to improve feeding habits. Additionally, close monitoring of centile charts and regular assessments for nutritional deficiencies is essential in the management of children with neurological disabilities. Involvement of a specialist paediatric dietician and implementation of a high-calorie diet with additional vitamin supplements is essential. Budden recommends frequent small feeds during the day with added carbohydrate foods to maintain growth. This is also shown to reduce agitation and irritability (Budden, 1997). Enteral tube feeding, such as nasogastric tubes and gastrostomy tubes, becomes necessary when a child cannot meet their nutritional or energy needs by oral feeding alone, or when there is a high risk of aspiration. Nasogastric or nasojejunal tubes are minimally invasive, and may be used for short-term nutritional support. They are unsuitable for long-term use because they can be easily dislodged, and can cause upper respiratory tract infections and intestinal perforation. For long-term enteral feeding, gastrostomy tube placement is required. Percutaneous endoscopic gastrostomy (PEG) placement is a minimally-invasive procedure and, once in place, allows for delivery of medications and high-calorie food in addition to oral intake, and reduces the risk of aspiration. It improves height and weight gain in girls with Rett syndrome, but does not completely reverse the growth failure that occurs (Motil et al., 2009). Minor complications include infections, stoma leakage, and tube dislodgement. Major complications include perforation, peritonitis and separation of the stomach from the abdominal wall (Marchand et al., 2006).

Other Clinical Considerations

In addition to treatment of specific symptomatology, it is important to take into account the overall functional effects of Rett syndrome. This requires extensive involvement of occupational therapy to improve the child's abilities and integrate her into every day family life. Speech and language therapy is needed to improve feeding and swallowing, and to improve communication. While girls with Rett syndrome usually display good non-verbal communication, the use of communication boards and switch devices may be employed to improve their ability to interact with their environments and express their needs (Weaving et al., 2005). Additionally, the use of alternative therapies such as music therapy and hydrotherapy is being explored. Music therapy can help relax the child and improve communication, attention, motivation and purposeful hand use in girls with Rett syndrome (Wigram et al., 2005). Hydrotherapy is thought to work by promoting relaxation, improving circulation, strengthening muscles and enhancing coordination, and therefore promote walking and restore mobility. One case study reports a reduction in stereotypic hand movements, improvement in feeding, improved walking balance and reduced anxiety and hyperactivity following 8 weeks of hydrotherapy (Bumin et al., 2003).

While these non-pharmacological therapies play a central role in the management of Rett syndrome, these girls syndrome frequently require multiple pharmacological interventions. Therefore, in order to minimise harm, pharmacovigilance is key. Given that they are predisposed to QT prolongation, medications that precipitate QT prolongation and cardiac arrhythmias should be avoided where possible, including pro-kinetic agents, antipsychotics (risperidone has the lowest risk of QT prolongation), tricyclic antidepressants and certain antimicrobials (such as erythromycin and ketoconazole) (Weaving et al., 2005). While β-blockers are the standard treatment for QT prolongation, one study suggests that they are not effective in the treatment of QT prolongation in MECP2-null mice, and that a sodium channel-blocker is a more suitable therapy in this case (McCauley et al., 2011). Additionally, since girls with Rett syndrome are usually on multiple different medications, strict knowledge of and monitoring for drug-drug interactions is required, particularly in cases where girls are taking anticonvulsant drugs that alter CYP450 metabolism.

In all, it is evident from the above that current management of Rett syndrome requires complex multidisciplinary input that must be integrated to ensure maximisation of the girl's functional abilities and minimisation of harm. However, as research into Rett syndrome grows, new treatments that target the core pathology are emerging.

Research into New Treatments

Though Rett syndrome was first described by Andrea Rett in 1960, it was only in 1999 that Rett syndrome was shown to be caused primarily by mutations of the MECP2 gene (Amir et al., 1999). More than 600 pathogenic MECP2 mutations have been identified, including nonsense, missense, frameshift and deletion mutations (Gardalla et al., 2011). The exact functions of MeCP2 remain unclear. It is involved in genome-wide transcriptional repression and global dampening of transcriptional noise (Nan et al., 1997). However, it may also be involved in selective transcriptional activation or enhancement (Chahrour et al., 2009), chromatin regulation (Nikitina et al., 2007A, B) and RNA processing (Young et al., 2005). MeCP2 is widely expressed in many cell types, and is particularly abundant in post-natal neurons (LaSalle et al., 2001). Its expression increases with increasing neuronal maturation (Shahbazian et al., 2002), reflecting its roles in CNS development, which include dendritic arborization and spine morphogenesis, acting through induction of neurotrophic factors such as Brain-Derived Neurotrophic Factor (BDNF) (Zhou et al., 2006).

Greater knowledge of the underlying biology allowed for the development of mouse models of Rett syndrome (Guy et al., 2001; Chen et al., 2001). These conditional MECP2 knockout mice undergo a period of normal development, followed by progressive neurological deterioration. Conditional deletion of MECP2 in post-mitotic neurons mimics the phenotype of *MECP2* knockout, indicating that it is MECP2 dysfunction in mature neurons that gives rise to the aberrant phenotype in Rett syndrome (Chen et al., 2001; Guy et al., 2001). Importantly, activation of the *MECP2* gene in MECP2 knockout mice is sufficient to reverse the phenotype (Guy et al., 2007; Giacometti et al., 2007). This demonstrated that neuronal function is not irreversibly impaired in Rett syndrome and that the course of the disease can be altered and is therefore amenable to treatment, even if treatment is given later in the course of the disease. Thus, while current management largely rests on symptom palliation and prevention using the strategies described above, the discovery that the disease process can be altered in Rett syndrome triggered new efforts to develop disease-modifying therapies that seek to alter the underlying pathogenesis.

In particular, there has been a surge in translational research using mouse models, seeking to identify molecular therapies that reverse the disease process in mouse models and which can be converted into viable therapies for human clinical trial.

These experimental therapies can be categorised into those that target the causative mutation, and those that target downstream function consequences of the genetic defect, including aberrant signalling pathways or dysfunctional neurotransmitter systems. Finally, given that our knowledge of the biology underlying Rett syndrome is still limited, several attempts are being made to exploit high throughput screening strategies to identify existing drug molecules that may be effective, as well as identify new cellular pathways affected by MECP2 mutations that may be targeted by existing treatments (these projects are listed at http://www.rsrt.org/researchers).

In short, recent progress in discovering the genetic basis of Rett syndrome, and the generation of mouse models that further our understanding of the pathophysiology and allow the development and testing of therapeutics, has ushered in a wave of new therapeutics at the pre-clinical and clinical stages of development. In light of this, this review aims to give a general overview of the progress made, by looking back on previous clinical trials that focused on Rett syndrome, before reviewing newer treatment strategies at both the clinical and preclinical stages that were largely developed with the use of mouse models (Figure 1).

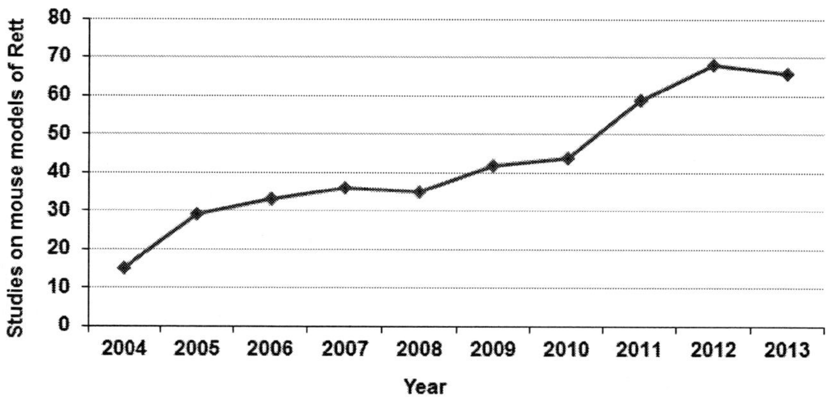

Figure 1. Estimated number of mouse studies of Rett syndrome in the past 10 years based on a pubmed search using the search words "Rett," "syndrome" and "mouse."

Previous Clinical Trials

Up until recently, clinical trials for Rett syndrome have been relatively few (Figure 2), and are listed in Table 1. In the pre-mutation era, trials for naltrexone, L-carnitine and the ketogenic diet were undertaken. Additionally, trials for FDA-approved medications that target specific symptoms of Rett syndrome, such as lamotrigine and bromocriptine, were trialled in Rett syndrome populations. Shortly after the discovery that Rett syndrome is caused by mutation of MeCP2, a key protein in DNA methylation, clinical trials for methyl donors folate and betaine, and creatine, were completed. The findings of these trials are summarised below (Table 1).

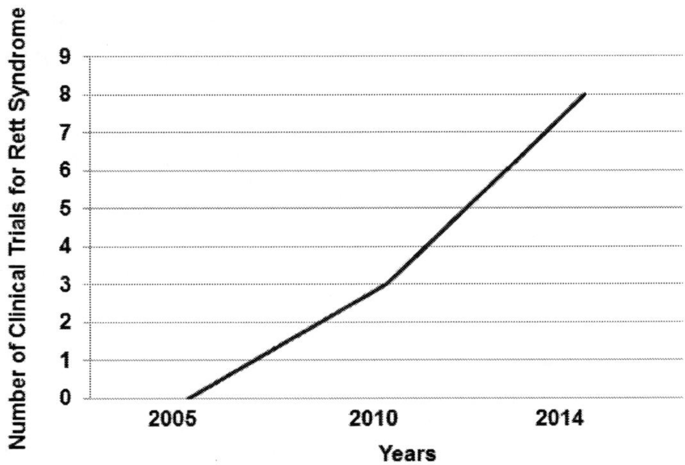

Figure 2. Estimated number of clinical trials in the past 10 years based on a pubmed search with "clinical trials" and the search words "Rett syndrome".

Table 1. A list of completed clinical trials performed in Rett syndrome populations

Ketogenic diet	(Haas et al., 1986)
Bromocriptine	(Zapella, 1990)
Naltrexone	(Percy et al., 1994)
Lamotrigine	(Stenborn et al., 1998)
Melatonin	(McArthur et al., 1998)
L-carnitine	(Ellaway et al., 1999)
Cerebrolysin	(Gorbachevskaya et al., 2001)
Vagus nerve stimulation	(Wilfong et al., 2006)
Folate and betaine	(Glaze et al., 2009)
Creatine	(Freilinger et al., 2011)
ω-3 polyunsaturated fatty acids	(De Felice et al., 2012)

In light of the prevalence of seizure disorders, the efficacy of lamotrigine in Rett syndrome populations was assessed in 1998, which demonstrated that patients respond well to lamotrigine. However, expansion of this study is required (Stenborn et al., 1998). Similarly, given that motor dysfuntion is prominent in Rett syndrome, the use of bromocriptine was assessed. While there were minor improvements in motor skills, there was no overall change in the disease state (Zapella, 1990).

Trials of naltrexone were conducted based on the findings of elevated β-endorphins in the cerebrospinal fluid and cerebral tissue of patients with Rett syndrome, and that intraventricular injection of endorphins into mice produced the clinical characteristics of Rett syndrome, which were reversible upon treatment with naltrexone (Percy, 2014). Naltrexone treatment caused improvement in breathing irregularities, such as a reduction in irregular breathing patterns, and an increase in minimum O_2 saturation levels and maximum CO_2 levels (Percy et al., 1994). However, this was likely due to the sedative effect of naltrexone. No improvement in behaviour, hand stereotypies, sleep parameters or seizure activity was noted, and it was suggested that naltrexone may have a negative effect on motor development and induce more rapid progression of the disorder. Similar findings were noted in a trial of naloxone (Glaze et al., 1989).

Studies have shown a functional deficiency of L-carnitine in Rett syndrome (Plochl et al., 1996). L-carnitine plays an important role in beta-fatty acid oxidation and mitochondrial energy production. Based on two case studies describing clinical improvement of various features of Rett syndrome following L-carnitine supplementation (Plochl et al., 1996) (Plioplys et al., 1996), a randomised-controlled trial investigating the efficacy of L-carnitine supplementation was performed. However, the clinical improvements were not as dramatic as those seen in these initial case studies. One trial showed subtle improvements in behavioural/social, orofacial/respiratory and apraxia scales, and overall patient well-being (Ellaway et al., 1999). Another trial showed a small but statistically significant improvement in sleep efficiency and energy levels, communication skills and expressive speech, and teeth-grinding (Ellaway et al., 2001). Six months of treatment with acetyl-L-carnitine was shown to increase heart rate variability, and therefore may reduce the risk of sudden death (Guideri et al., 2005). The overall impact on the disease was minor and no long-term studies examining the efficacy of L-carnitine have been reported.

Trials for folate supplementation are based on two sets of findings. Firstly, analysis of CSF in RTT patients found reduced levels of the folate derivative,

5-methyltetrahydrofolate (Ormazabal et al., 2005). Following the discovery that mutations in MeCP2 are the genetic basis of Rett syndrome, causing impaired or absent binding of MeCP2 to methyl-cytosine in the promotor region of genes and subsequent impairment of transcriptional repression, clinical trials assessing the use of methyl group donors, folate and betaine, were conducted. This is based on the hypothesis that increased cytosine methylation through exogenous administration of methyl group donors could enhance MeCP2 binding (Percy, 2002). While subjective improvements in behaviour were observed, no objective evidence of clinical improvement was reported (Glaze et al., 2009; Hagebeuk et al., 2009). Further trials for folic acid supplementation have reported no improvements (Hagebeuk et al., 2011; Hageburg et al., 2012).

Clinical trials for creatine supplementation were developed based on the similar hypothesis that DNA methylation in the presence of a faulty MeCP2 protein may be maximised by increasing endogenous levels of methyl groups. About 80 % of labile methyl groups generated through the re-methylation cycle are used for the synthesis of creatine. Thus, creatine supplementation can increase availability of labile methyl groups for other reactions such as DNA methylation. Clinical trials showed a statistically significant increase in global methylation. While improvements in motor and behavioural assessments were noted, these were not statistically significant (Freilinger et al., 2011).

While the beneficial effects of the ketogenic diet in refractory epilepsy have been widely assessed (Keane et al., 2006; Neal et al., 2008; Dressler et al., 2010), its impact on other features of Rett syndrome has not been established. Haas et al (1986) performed an uncontrolled study assessing the effect of the ketogenic diet in 7 girls with Rett syndrome. He reported improved seizure control, but only minor improvements in behavioural and motor abilities in 5 girls after 3 months. Since then, no further clinical trials have been performed. A case study in 2003 reported the effects of a 4-year ketogenic diet in a child with Rett syndrome, which included a reduction in seizure frequency that was greater than that achieved by anticonvulsant medication, and subjective improvement in concentration, behaviour and language (Leibhaber et al., 2003).

While the ketogenic diet causes moderate changes in the clinical severity of Rett syndrome, another dietary intervention has also been assessed; supplementation with ω-3-polyunsaturated fatty acids. One placebo-controlled study on 20 girls reported significant improvements in motor function, non-verbal communication and breathing abnormalities and a decrease in the levels of markers of oxidative stress (De Felice et al., 2012). However, these results have not been further substantiated.

While the majority of cases of epilepsy in Rett syndrome respond to anti-epileptic medication, there are cases of treatment resistant, for which vagus nerve stimulation has undergone clinical trial. Unmatched trial of vagus nerve stimulation in 7 girls who had previously failed two trials of antiepileptic therapy demonstrated its safety and efficacy, with over 50% reduction in seizure frequency in 6 out of 7 girls.

An additional open pilot study of the brain-derived peptidergic drug cerebrolysis was performed on 9 girls with Rett syndrome. It reported improved motor function, behavioural activity, attention and non-verbal communication, along with a change of EEG parameters towards normal values. However, further studies of cerebrolysin therapy have not been reported (Gorbachevskaya et al., 2001).

Finally, as described above, a trial of exogenous melatonin for treatment of sleep disturbance in Rett syndrome was performed, which showed reductions in sleep onset latency (McArthur et al., 1999).

It is evident form the above that, other than investigations of certain established medical treatments such as lamotrigine and melatonin for treatment of specific symptoms, clinical trials for Rett syndrome have yielded few results. These trials were largely based on small studies of clinical findings in Rett syndrome patients. However, with the development of mouse models of Rett syndrome, knowledge of the underlying pathophysiology has grown, and allowed for the identification of new drug targets in the disease process.

New Therapeutic Strategies

As said, the development of mouse models of Rett syndrome has stimulated efforts to develop and experimentally validate new treatment strategies for this complex neurodevelopmental disorder (Figure 2). Presently, the first products of this new wave in translational research are now reaching clinical trial, and are listed in Table 2. These treatments target a variety of putative disease processes in Rett syndrome, including BDNF dysregulation, glutamate excitotoxicity, serotonin dysfunction, norepinephrine dysfunction and oxidative damage. They are described according to their believed mechanism of action below. In general, current treatment strategies for Rett syndrome are based either on restoration of gene function, correction of aberrant BDNF signalling, and alteration of dysregulated neurotransmitter systems. Even newer strategies focus on glial dysfunction, or alteration of other signalling pathways thought to be modified in Rett syndrome, such cholesterol biosynthesis. These are summarised below.

Table 2. Drug treatments currently under clinical trial for Rett syndrome

Glatiramer acetate	ClinicalTrials.gov Identifier: NCT02023424 ClinicalTrials.gov Identifier: NCT02153723
Fingolimod	ClinicalTrials.gov Identifier: NCT02061137
EPI-743	ClinicalTrials.gov Identifier: NCT01822249
Recombinant human IGF-1	ClinicalTrials.gov Identifier: NCT02061137
NNZ-2566	ClinicalTrials.gov Identifier: NCT01703533
Desipramine	ClinicalTrials.gov Identifier: NCT00990691
Dextromethorphan	ClinicalTrials.gov Identifier: NCT01520363

Translational Research: Targeting the Gene

As stated above, one line of translational research is investigation of therapies that target the causative genetic defect, restoring MECP2 function through a number of different strategies, including reactivation of the normal allele, gene therapy, or aminoglycoside treatment.

MECP2 is located on the X chromosome, and is therefore subject to X chromosome inactivation (XCI), whereby one of the X chromosomes in each cell undergoes epigenetic silencing by DNA methylation. Therefore, each cell expresses either the normal allele only, or the mutant allele only. Reactivation of the normal MECP2 allele is theoretically possible. Initial studies used treatment with 5-azacytadine, a chemical compound known to reduce genomic methylation levels (Mohandas et al., 1981). However, the risk is that other genes on the X chromosome are also reactivated, leading to the X-linked gene dosage problem for which XCI evolved. There are a number of groups currently using high-throughput screening methods to identify different compounds that could reactivate MECP2 function, and these are listed on http://www.rsrt.org/research/our-projects.

Another method for restoring MECP2 function is gene therapy, involving systemic delivery of an intact *MECP2* gene using the adenovirus-associated virus 9 (AAV9) as a vehicle. This resulted in widespread distribution and physiological levels of Mecp2 protein in the brain, and increased neuronal size and brain weight compared to untreated controls. Furthermore, treatment caused improvements in survival and motor function in mice models compared to controls, but did not affect respiratory function (Garg et al., 2013). An issue associated with gene therapy is dosage, as overexpression of *MECP2* also causes neurological dysfunction in both humans and mouse models (Meins et al., 2005) (Van Esch et al., 2005) (Luikenhuis et al., 2004). Girls with Rett syndrome are mosaic, and therefore gene therapy would lead to overexpression of *MECP2* in cells that express the normal allele. Thus, while high viral titres are necessary to achieve widespread transfection of target tissues, having more than one copy of the gene in any cell would cause harm. This is one of the many issues surrounding gene therapy that must be overcome before it can become a safe therapeutic option.

Restoration of *MECP2* expression may be achieved in cases where the causative mutation is a nonsense mutation associated with premature stop codons (PSCs) by treatment with aminoglycoside antibiotics. These antibiotics permit ribosomal read-through of PSCs, which facilitates complete transcription of the gene and subsequent generation of a full-length functional protein. This strategy is already being employed for treatment of Duchenne muscular dystrophy and Cystic Fibrosis (Gardalla et al., 2011). Given that up to 35% cases of typical Rett syndrome are caused by nonsense mutations (Brendel et al., 2011), aminoglycosides are a promising possibility. Production of full-length Mecp2 protein was observed following gentamycin treatment in *in vitro* studies, though readthrough efficiency varies (Brendel et al., 2009; Popescu et al., 2010; Brendel et al., 2011). Chronic gentamycin treatment carries a significant risk of ototoxicity and nephrotoxicity. Therefore related compounds with reduced toxicity are currently under development, including PTC124 and NB54 (Welch et al., 2007; Nudelman et al., 2009).

However, it is important to note that none of these innovative strategies are near the point of translation for human clinical trials. They require further development and characterisation in mouse models before their use in Rett syndrome can be assessed in human subjects.

Translational Research: Targeting Factors Downstream of MECP2 Function

Aberrant Neurotrophism

Much research has focused on activating factors that act downstream of MeCP2. MeCP2 binds widely across the genome, and has complex roles in transcriptional activation and repression, methylation repression, chromatin remodelling and regulation of non-coding RNAs (Castro et al., 2014). One well-established target of MeCP2 is Brain-Derived Neurotrophic Factor (BDNF), a factor that is important for neuronal development, synaptic maturation and plasticity (Li et al., 2014). BDNF acts through Trkb receptors to activate a number of signalling cascades, including MAPK, PI3K and PSD-95 pathways, and influence neuronal maturation and synaptic plasticity.

Many animal studies demonstrate that MECP2 modulates BDNF expression. Its expression in the brain is low during post-natal development, and rises during post-natal development, correlating with MECP2 activity in the developing brain. In mouse models of Rett syndrome, BDNF expression is normal during pre-symptomatic phase in the first 3-4 weeks of life, but declines as the Rett-like phenotype develops (Chang et al., 2006; Wang et al., 2006). At 5-6 weeks, BDNF expression is lower in the cerebellum and brainstem compared to wild-type mice (Wang et al., 2006; Ogier et al., 2007; Kline et al., 2010). By 7 weeks, all areas of the brain show lower BDNF expression in MECP2 mutant mice (Chang et al., 2006; Schmid et al., 2012). Additionally, BDNF deletion in postnatal forebrain excitatory neurons recapitulates many of the neurological symptoms of MECP2 knockout mice, such as hind limb clasping, reduced brain weight and smaller olfactory and hippocampal neurons (Chang et al., 2006). However, more evidence is required regarding BDNF expression levels in patients with Rett syndrome, as CSF and autopsy studies are contradictory. While CSF studies suggest that BDNF levels in Rett patients are comparable to unaffected individuals, brain autopsies indicate reduced levels of BDNF (Li et al., 2014).

Restoration of BDNF expression in mouse models of Rett syndrome has been shown to attenuate the disease process. BDNF overexpression in the forebrain neurons of MECP2-null mice extended lifespan, improved locomotion, increased brain weight, and reduced spontaneous neuronal firing (Chang et al., 2006). Similarly, BDNF overexpression in hippocampal neurons *in vitro* reversed the dendritic atrophy caused by MECP2 knockdown (Larimore et al., 2009). However, the clinical utility of BDNF is limited by its inability to cross the blood-brain barrier (BBB). Therefore, different strategies have been employed to upregulate BDNF signalling by pharmacological manipulation.

Insulin-like growth factor (IGF-1) is also involved in neuronal survival and maturation (D'Ercole et al., 1996), and similarly activates the MAPK, PI3K and PSD-95 signalling pathways activated by BDNF (Zheng et al., 2004). Importantly, IGF-1 can cross the BBB, particularly in its tri-peptide form, (1-3)IGF-1. Treatment of mouse models of Rett syndrome with injections of either full-length IGF-1 or the tripeptide form, (1-3)IGF-1, increases expression of markers for synaptic transmission (Corvin et al., 2012) and produces a partial reversal of the phenotype, with improvements in locomotor, cardiac and respiratory function, and an increase in life expectancy (Tropea et al., 2009; Castro et al., 2014). Importantly, full length recombinant human IGF-1 is already licensed for clinical use in the paediatric population for the treatment of growth deficits. This allowed for rapid progression to human clinical trials. A safety assessment in six girls with Rett syndrome demonstrated its tolerability, and reported that subtle clinical improvements, reflected by a reduction in the International Severity Scale and subjective reports of cognitive and motor skill improvement, occurred during the 6 months of treatment (Pini et al., 2012). These benefits regress upon cessation of IGF-1 treatment (Pini et al., 2014). An advanced phase 2, double-blind, placebo-controlled trial of full length rhIGF-1 (Mecasermin) is ongoing (ClinicalTrials.gov Identifier: NCT01777542). Additionally, NNZ-2566 is a synthetic analogue of a the (1-3)IGF-1 tripeptide. It is also undergoing clinical trial for treatment of Fragile X syndrome, Rett syndrome and traumatic brain injury, and is in the second phase of clinical trial for Rett syndrome (ClinicalTrials.gov Identifier: NCT01703533).

Fingolimod is a sphinosine-1 phosphate receptor modulator developed for the treatment of multiple sclerosis. It increases BDNF expression via activation of the ERK signalling pathway. In cultured neurons, fingolimod increases BDNF levels and counteracts NMDA-mediated neuronal death in a BDNF-dependent manner. Treatment of MECP2-null mice caused increased brain levels of BDNF, and improved locomotor function (Deogracias et al., 2012). Based on these results, a phase 1 clinical trial is underway to determine the safety of oral fingolimod in children with Rett syndrome, as well as assess whether it increases endogenous levels of BDNF in human subjects (ClinicalTrials.gov Identifier: NCT02061137).

Glatiramer acetate is another drug that was developed for the treatment of multiple sclerosis. Also like fingolimod, the hypothetical basis for its use in Rett syndrome is its effect on BDNF levels in the brain. It has been shown to increase BDNF levels in both MS patients and mouse models of Rett syndrome (Ben-Zeev et al., 2011). It is now undergoing two open-label clinical trials assessing its safety and its impact on various aspects of the Rett syndrome phenotype (ClinicalTrials.gov Identifier: NCT02023424, NCT02153723).

Other therapies targeting BDNF signalling that aim to ameliorate the respiratory difficulties observed in Rett syndrome have also been investigated in mouse models, though these have yet to reach translation to human clinical trials.

There is a significant reduction in BDNF expression in the brainstem and nodose cranial sensory ganglia in mouse models of Rett syndrome, which are structures critical for cardiorespiratory control. The ampakine drug CX546 is a positive modulator of glutaminergic AMPA receptors that is known to increase activity-dependent BDNF expression by neuronal activation. In Mecp2-null mice, treatment with CX546 increased the BDNF content of nodose cranial sensory ganglia by 42%. Additionally, treatment caused improvements in respiratory function by restoration of breathing frequency (Ogier et al., 2007).

Another example are BDNF "mimetics," which are Trkb receptor agonists that are capable of crossing the BBB. They include LM22A-4 and 7,8-DHF, and they have been shown to increase survival and body mass, improve motor and respiratory function and increase neuronal size (Johnson et al., 2012; Schmid et al., 2012).

An alternative method to increase endogenous levels of BDNF is by Environmental Enrichment (EE). Environmental approaches may alter cellular pathology by epigenetic mechanisms. Kondo et al., (2008) demonstrated modest elevation of cerebellar BDNF levels in heterozygous MECP2+/- female mice (but not MECP2-null male mice), and reduced motor incoordination following exposure to a rich and stimulating environment. Nag et al (2009) reported an improvement in motor coordination, locomotion and learning. The findings of improved motor function were reinforced by Lonetti et al., (2010).

Finally, the use of deep brain stimulation and transmagnetic stimulation for treatment of Rett syndrome are under assessment. Known to increase endogenous levels of BDNF (Hamani et al., 2012) and promote hippocampal neurogenesis and dendritic complexity in mouse models of Rett syndrome, its effect on cognition is currently under investigation in the Zoghbi lab, funded by RSRT.

Overall, BDNF has proved a promising drug target in the development of disease-modifying therapies for the treatment of Rett syndrome. It has generated four treatments currently under clinical trial in human subjects: IGF-1, NNZ- 2566, fingolimod and glatiramer acetate. Two of these (IGF-1 and NNZ-2566) were originally developed in mouse models.

For a list of the Clinical Trials currently on-going see Table 3.

Table 3. Experimental treatments for Rett syndrome currently undergoing human clinical trials (as listed in ClinicalTrials.gov website)

Drug Name	ClinicalTrials.gov Identifier	Phase	Summary of outcome measures
Glatiramer acetate	NCT02023424	1	1. Measure effect on eleptiform activity on EEG 2. Observe effect on clinical phenotype and bodily development 3. Incidence of adverse effects
	NCT02153723	2	1. Measure effect on gait speed 2. Measure effect on sleep parameters 3. Measure effect on respiratory dysfunction 4. Measure changes on EEG 5. Assess impact on quality of life using Child Health Questionnaire.
Fingolimod	NCT02061137	2	1. Blood and CSF levels of BDNF following treatment
EPI-743	NCT01822249	2	1. Rett Syndrome Clinical Severity Score after 6 months measuring disease progression. 2. Oxidative stress biomarkers 3. Head circumference 4. Rett Syndrome Behavioural Questionnaire 5. Respiratory Disturbance Index by polysomnography
Recombinant human IGF-1	NCT01777542	2	1. Rett Syndrome Behavioural Questionnaire 2. Quantitative measures of respiration 3. Evaluation of cortical function using visual evoked potentials
NNZ-2566 (1-3)IGF-1 analogue	NCT01703533	2	1. Incidence of adverse events 2. Changes in EEG activity 3. Motor Behavioural Assessment 4. Clinical Severity Scale 5. Aberrant Behaviour Checklist 6. Adaptive Behaviour Scale 7. Clinical Global Impression of Severity 8. Changes in physiological parameters
Desipramine	NCT00990691	2	1. Observe effect on respiratory disturbances
Dextromethorphan	NCT01520363	2	1. Neuropsychological testing (Mullens Scale of Early Learning). 2. Behavioural assessment (Vineland Adaptive Behaviour Scales)

Dysfunctional Neurotransmission

Defects in numerous neurotransmitter systems have been observed in Rett syndrome, in both animal models and in patients, including the 5-HT, noradrenaline, dopamine, acetylcholine, GABA and glutamine systems.

The Biogenic Amines: Noradrenaline, Dopamine and Serotonin Deficits in Rett Syndrome

Samaco et al., (2008) demonstrated that levels of aminergic neurotransmitter metabolites, HVA and5-HIAA are reduced in patients with Rett syndrome, and confirmed this in MECP2$^{null/y}$ mice. They also found a reduction in the levels of synthetic enzymes for these neurotransmitters, and demonstrated that MECP2 is involved in regulation of these enzymes. Ide et al., (2005) showed progressive deficiency in amine neurotransmitters in the whole brains of MECP2 null mice that increased with each post-natal day. These findings are reflected in post-mortem studies of Rett syndrome brains (Brucke et al., 1987; Lekman et al., 1989). Deregulation of these neurotransmitter systems has been implicated in a wide variety of clinical manifestations of Rett syndrome.

For example, norepinephrine deficiency has been linked to respiratory dysfunction in Rett syndrome. Studies show catecholamine deficits in the brainstem, chamoafferent and sympathoadrenergic systems and the locus ceruleus of MECP2 deficient mice (Viemari et al., 2005; Roux et al., 2008; Roux et al., 2010). Additionally, neurons containing tysoine hydroxylase, the rate-limiting enzyme in norepinephrine and dopamine synthesis, are reduced in both central and peripheral nuclei (Roux et al., 2008; Roux et al., 2010). A proof of principle study showed that the rhythm produced by an isolated respiratory network within brainstem slices from MECP2null mice was stabilised by exogenous treatment with norepinephrine (Viemari et al., 2005). Subsequently, MECP2-deficient mice were treated with desipramine, a tricyclic antidepressant that, in particular, inhibits norepinephrine uptake. It increased the number of TH-containing neurons, improved breathing rhythm and increased the lifespan of MECP2null mice, though levels of norepinephrine were not altered (Roux et al., 2007; Zanella et al., 2008). The effect of desipramine on the respiratory irregularities in patients with Rett syndrome is currently undergoing a phase 2 clinical trial with an expected completion date of September 2014 (ClinicalTrials.gov Identifier: NCT00990691).

Deficiencies in serotonin (5-HT) transmission are also thought to play a role in the pathogenesis of breathing dysfunction in Rett syndrome. Serotonin stimulates ventilation in response to CO_2 (Richardson et al., 2004) and treatment of MECP2 mutant mice with citalopram improves CO_2 chemosensitivity (Toward et al., 2013). Additionally, activation of serotonergic neurons via 5-HT1A receptors is involved in termination of respiration (Kerr et al., 1999). The 5-HT1A agonist, buspirone, was used to effectively treat post-operative apneusis (Wilken et al., 1997), and abnormal breathing in Rett syndrome (Andaku et al., 2005). The 5-HT1A agonist, F15599, corrects apnoea and breathing irregularity in multiple mouse models of Rett syndrome (Levitt et al., 2013), and has undergone a phase 1 of a clinical trial as NLX-101 by Neurolixis in healthy volunteers.

Serotonin dysfunction is also thought to play a role in the sympatho-parasympathetic imbalance that occurs in Rett syndrome. Reduced vagal drive and therefore unopposed sympathetic stimulation of the cardiovascular system increases the risk of cardiac arrhythmias, excessive swings in heart rate and blood pressure, reduced heart rate variability and sudden death (Kerr et al., 1997; Richter et al., 2003). Reduced heart rate variability correlates with reduced levels of serotonin (Guideri et al., 2004). Deletion of the 5-HT1A receptors in mouse models increased susceptibility to sudden death at times of stress (Carnevali et al., 2012). Treatment with a 5-HT1A agonist disinhibited the vagal neurons (Chen et al., 2008). This may be an added benefit for 5-HT1A agonist treatment of Rett syndrome.

Serotonin is also implicated in mood disorders, including anxiety, depression and obsessive compulsive disorder. Therefore, serotonin dysfunction may underlie the mood disturbance and hand stereotypies that occurs in Rett syndrome. Furthermore, the anxiety and mood disorder observed in Rett patients is thought to exacerbate breathing dysfunction (Abdala et al., 2014). The selective serotonin reuptake inhibitors (SSRIs) citalopram and fluoxetine are effective for treatment of mood disturbance, but not repetitive behaviours, in Rett syndrome (King et al., 2009; Chapleau et al., 2013; Williams et al., 2013). While 5-HT levels are rapidly restored following treatment with SSRIs, their antidepressant effect take up to 3 weeks to occur. This suggests that it is not simply the levels of 5-HT in the brain, but its long-term effect on synaptic and neuronal function, that exerts the effect on mood disturbance. In particular, the role of serotonin in circuit maturation has been studied in the pathogenesis of mood disorder in Rett syndrome. The post-natal period during which Rett syndrome develops is considered a key period in the maturation of anxiety circuits (Leonardo et al., 2008). There is increasing evidence that serotonin function is important during the developmental period for the maturation of anxiety-related circuits (Leonardo et al., 2008). Studies of 5-HT1A receptor knockout mice demonstrate that decreased expression of 5-HT1A receptors during the development caused increased anxiety, which can be reversed by restoring 5-HT1A receptor expression during the early postnatal period (Gross et al., 2002). This suggests that neurodevelopmental disruption of 5-HT1A receptor expression may play a role in the pathogenesis of anxiety in Rett syndrome. Therefore, 5-HT1A agonists may not only be effective for treatment of anxiety in Rett syndrome, but may serve a protective effect against the onset of anxiety if given early in the course of the disease. In particular, specificity for post-synaptic 5-HT1A receptors is thought to enhance the antidepressant effect, as concurrent inhibition of presynaptic 5-HT1A receptors in the dorsal raphe nuclei is shown to strengthen antidepressant action in animal studies (Newmand-Tancredi et al., 2009). While current 5-HT1A agonists such as buspirone lack specificity and potency, newer 5-HT1A agonists such as NLX-101 show high 5-HT1A agonist efficacy and specificity for post-synaptic 5-HT1A receptors (Newman-Tancredi et al., 2009; Abdala et al., 2014), and have demonstrated anti-depressant-like properties in mouse models of depression (Assie et al., 2010). Finally, these newer 5-HT1A agonists with post-synaptic specificity are shown to increase dopamine levels in the frontal cortex (Newman-Tancredi et al., 2010), and they are currently undergoing clinical trials for the treatment of Parkinson's disease (Abdala et al., 2014).

The role of serotonin in circuit maturation during the post-natal period is not restricted to anxiety-related circuits (Leonardo et al., 2008). Its role in somatosensory circuits has also been demonstrated (Fox et al., 1992; Nakamura et al., 2006). Therefore, long-term treatment with 5-HT1À agonists may have far-reaching benefits on brain function in Rett syndrome. Additionally, direct injection of the SSRI, fluoxetine, into normal rat brains has been shown to induce Mecp2 at both the mRNA and protein level (Cassell et al., 2006). This further implicates the potential of serotonin-modulating therapy in the treatment of Rett syndrome, as there are suggestions that early treatment with fluoxetine to induce MECP2 expression could modify the course of the disease (Pan et al., 2012).

In conclusion, given that these new potent and highly specific 5-HT1A agonists such as NLX-101 have been shown to possess pro-motor effects in rats with dopaminergic lesions, potent antidepressant effects (Assie et al., 2010), precognitive activity (Depoortere et al., 2010), and the capacity to reverse the respiratory phenotype in mouse models of Rett syndrome (Levitt et al., 2013), their show great promise in improving the symptoms of Rett syndrome.

Acetylcholine Deficits in Rett Syndrome

Acetylcholine (Ach) is another neurotransmitter that shows alterations in Rett syndrome. Studies show reduced acetylcholine transferase activity and reduced vesamicol binding to vesicular actylcholine transporters (Wenk et al., 1996). This led to the hypothesis that choline supplementation may boost Ach synthesis and thereby improve brain cholinergic function. MECP2null mice were given choline supplementation early in post-natal development, which caused subtle improvements in motor function and locomotion (Nag et al., 2007). This may be due to increased nerve growth factors levels in the striatum (Nag et al., 2008). The acetylcholine esterase inhibitor, donepezil, has been proposed as a potential therapy though, to date, no formal clinical trials have been completed.

Excitatory/Inhibitory Imbalance: Dysfunctional Glutamate and GABA Transmission in Rett Syndrome

In addition to the biogenic amines, dysfunctional glutamate and GABA transmission has also been implicated in the pathogenesis of Rett syndrome, because of neurophysiological studies showing excitatory/inhibitory imbalances in MECP2 mutant mice. However, unlike the alterations in biogenic amine activity, there is no clear cut pattern to the changes in GABA and glutamate transmission in Rett syndrome mouse models. Variations in GABA and glutamate activity are regional and age-dependent (El-Khoury et al., 2014).

There is impairment of long-term plasticity, and in general there appears to be increased excitatory synaptic transmission in the brainstem and hippocampus, and decreased excitatory transmission in the somatosensory and motor-frontal cortices (El-Khoury et al., 2014).

In the brainstem of MECP2-deficient mice, there is reduced quantal release of GABA, reduced expression of pre-synaptic GABA transporters and impaired function of post-synaptic $GABA_A$ receptors, leading to inhibitory-excitatory imbalance (Medrihan et al, 2008). This may contribute to the respiratory dysfunction observed in Rett syndrome, as treatment with the GABA reuptake blocker, tiagabine, increased the lifespan of MECP2-deficient mice (El-Khoury et al., 2014), while combination of a GABA modulator with a 5-HT1A agonist improved respiratory function in MECP2 heterozygous mice (Abdala et al., 2010). Similarly, treatment with the fast-acting benzodiazepine, midazolam, produced transient improvements breathing irregularities, with a reduction in apnoea and apneusis (Voituron et al., 2011).

In line with this evidence of GABA dysfunction in Rett syndrome, another group showed that selective removal of MECP2 from GABAergic neurons produced many of the autistic features of Rett syndrome, including repetitive behaviours. These MeCP2-deficiency GABAergic neurons show reduced inhibitory quantal size (Chao et al., 2010). These studies imply a role for therapies that enhance GABA transmission in the treatment of Rett syndrome.

The hippocampus shows increased excitatory transmission (Moretti et al., 2006; El-Khoury et al., 2014), and impaired long-term plasticity (Asaka et al., 2006). One study shows a simultaneous decrease in GABA and glutamate content in the hippocampus (El-Khoury et al., 2014). There is reduced spontaneous firing and excitatory postsynaptic current (EPSC) amplitude, and subtle alterations in the excitatory/inhibitory balance in CA3 hippocampal circuitry, rendering the hippocampal network hyperexcitable (Zhang et al., 2008; Calfa et al., 2011). There are reports of reductions in excitable synaptic connectivity in hippocampal neurons (Chao et al., 2007), which correlates with anatomic evidence of reduced dendritic branching in MECP2null neurons.

Conversely, there is decreased excitatory activity in the somatosensory and motor-frontal cortices. Studies of layer 5 pyramidal neurons in the somatosensory cortex showed reduced spontaneous excitatory synaptic input and smaller miniature excitatory postsynaptic current amplitude, which is attributed to impaired glutaminergic synaptic transmission (Dani et al., 2005). These reductions in excitatory synaptic activity, linked to reduced quantal release at the synapse, and overall reduced excitatory connectivity, are thought to contribute to the impairment of LTP induction (Dani et al., 2009). Similarly, studies of circuits in the motor-frontal cortex showed reduced excitatory synaptic input following localised knockdown of MECP2 (Wood et al., 2009; Wood et al., 2010).

Thus, though results are divergent, what is evident is that there is altered excitatory-inhibitory transmission in the brains of people with Rett syndrome (Medrihan et al., 2008) (El-Khoury et al., 2014). This implicates glutamate and GABA transmission modulators as potential treatments for Rett syndrome. While GABA reuptake blockers and benzodiazepines are being assessed for treatment of respiratory dysfunction, modulators of glutamate function are being investigated for a wide range of effects. For instance, as mentioned above, the AMPA receptor agonist CX546 has been investigated for treatment of breathing dysfunction in mouse models of Rett syndrome by increasing BDNF levels through neuronal activation (Ogier et al., 2007). Conversely,

NDMA receptor antagonists are being tested for treatment of Rett syndrome on the basis that glutamate-mediated excitotoxicity may contribute to the pathogenesis of Rett syndrome. This is supported by studies of glial dysfunction in Rett syndrome, which find abnormal glutamate clearance by astrocytes and increased glutamate synthesis by microglia in mouse models of Rett syndrome (Maezawa et al., 2010; Okabe et al., 2012). *In vitro* experiments for memantine showed reversal of impaired plasticity in Mecp2-hippocampal tissue, but this was not backed up by *in vivo* studies (Weng et al., 2011). Based on findings of elevated concentrations in glutatmate in the CSF of patients with Rett syndrome (Hamberger et al., 1992; Lappalainen et al., 1996), increased NMDA receptor density in the frontal cortex (Blue et al., 1999), and overall heightened synaptic cycling of glutamate in younger girls with Rett syndrome (Naidu et al., 2001), the dextromethorphan NMDA antagonist is currently undergoing phase 2 placebo-controlled clinical trial to assess whether blocking this toxic neuronal stimulation may cause improvements in cognitive function (Gardalla et al., 2011) (ClinicalTrials.gov Identifier: NCT01520363).

Glial Dysfunction

MECP2 is known to play a role in neuronal development including synaptogenesis, dendritic branching and electrophysiological responses. Additionally, reactivation of MECP2 in neurons can rescue the Rett syndrome phenotype. Therefore, up until recently, it was thought that Rett syndrome resulted exclusively from MECP2 loss in neurons. However, it was subsequently found that astrocytes in MECP2 mutant mice failed to support neuronal morphology *in vitro* (Ballas et al., 2009). It was then shown that in MECP2null mice, restoration of MECP2 function in astrocytes caused improvement in aspects of the disease phenotype, including locomotion, anxiety levels, irregular breathing patterns and lifespan, leading the group to conclude that astrocytic dysfunction in Rett syndrome contributes to disease progression (Lioy et al., 2011). Further study shows that MECP2 deletion in astrocytes leads to dysfunctional clearance of glutamate (Okabe et al., 2012). Studies comparing the effect of the culture medium of MCP2-deficiency astrocytes and microglia showed that the medium derived from MECP2-deficient microglia was neurotoxic, while the medium from MECP2-deficient astrocytes was not. The toxic component was identified as glutamate, as the MECP2-deficient microglia showed a 5-fold increase in extracellular glutamate levels, causing neuronal toxicity, due to increased glutamate synthesis and release by microglia. This neurotoxicity was counteracted by treatment with glutamate receptor antagonists (Maezawa et al., 2010).

Therefore, microglia is implicated in the pathogenesis of Rett syndrome through increased secretion of neurotoxic glutamate (Maezawa et al., 2010). Additionally, it is now thought that their phagocytic function plays a role in removal of toxic debris, CNS development and synaptic pruning, and that loss of this function contributes to the pathogenesis of Rett syndrome (Derecki et al., 2013). Bone marrow transplantation following irradiation-mediated immune ablation in 4 week-old MECP2-null mice caused microglial engraftment, which halted disease progression, improved many aspects of the phenotype including breathing irregularities, motor dysfunction and behavioural dysfunction, and increased the lifespan from 8 weeks to 1 year. Similarly, reactivation of MECP2 in myeloid cells halted disease progression, and treatment with the pharmacological inhibitor of phagocytosis annexin eliminated the benefit and caused a build-up of apoptopic CNS debris. This suggests that impaired phagocytic clearance by microglia is important in the underlying neuropathology of Rett syndrome (Derecki et al., 2012). However, these results have not been repeated.

Oxidative Stress

Numerous studies have linked Mecp2 deficiency to increased levels of oxidative stress (OS) markers in both patients with Rett syndrome and MECP2 mutant mouse models (De Felice et al., 2012; De Felice et al., 2014). Additionally, the degree of oxidative stress-mediated neuronal damage has been shown to correlate with the extent of Mecp2 dysfunction and the phenotypic severity. In light of these findings, the use of ω-3 polyunsaturated fatty acid supplementation was assessed in patients with Rett syndrome, because of their antioxidant properties. One placebo-controlled study on 20 girls reported significant improvements in motor function, non-verbal communication and breathing abnormalities and a decrease in the levels of markers of oxidative stress (De Felice et al., 2012). Furthermore, a phase 2 clinical trial is underway investigating the efficacy of EPI-743 for the treatment of Rett syndrome (ClinicalTrials.gov Identifier: NCT01822249). EPI-743 is a vitamin E-based para-benzoquinone therapeutic with proven efficacy in the treatment of disorders characterised by oxidative stress (Enns et al., 2012). Initially developed for the treatment of mitochondrial disorders, its use in the treatment of Rett syndrome is now being assessed.

New Lines of Investigation

As funding for research in Rett syndrome grows, new methods are being used to more rapidly identify promising drug treatments and hasten their progression to clinical trial. *In vivo* screening strategies are being employed to identify existing drugs and small molecules that show efficacy in amelioration of symptoms in mouse models. Carried out by the Zoghbi lab in Baylor College of Medicine, and the Pieper lab in University of Texas, these projects are listed on the RSRT website. High-throughput screening is also being used to identify compounds that reactivate the normal MECP2 allele in mouse cells. Additionally, high throughput screening strategies are being employed to identify new drug targets for which drugs can be developed for treatment of Rett syndrome, by identification of genetic modifiers that impact on the severity of the disease. In one study that employed a mutagenesis screen in *MECP2*null mice, five supressors that ameliorated MECP2 loss were identified. One of these suppressors was a stop codon mutation in *Sqle*, which codes for squalene epoxidase, a rate limiting enzyme in cholesterol biosynthesis. This suppressor reduced the symptoms of Rett syndrome in mouse models. This suggests that downregulation of cholesterol biosynthesis can improve symptoms in Rett syndrome. Subsequent examination of lipid profiles in non-suppressed $MECP2^{null}$ males showed significant abnormalities in the liver and brain. These abnormalities, along with some motor abnormalities, were ameliorated by treatment with statins and lifespan was increased (Buchovecky et al., 2013). These experiments require repetition in other mouse models before moving on to human clinical trials. This study highlights that, as research into therapies for Rett syndrome grows, more and more diverse cellular pathways are becoming implicated in its pathogenesis.

Conclusion

From the above, it is evident that a wide range of different approaches to modifying the disease process in Rett syndrome are currently under investigation, from stimulation of neurotrophic factors, to correction of deregulated neurotransmitter systems, to correction of oxidative stress in Rett syndrome. Furthermore, this review highlights the many more innovative strategies currently under development, from X chromosome inactivation to gene therapy, environmental enrichment to deep brain stimulation, haematopoietic stem cell transplantation to dietary supplementation. Research into Rett syndrome has led to many exciting discoveries in the field of human neurodevelopment, and has implicated a diverse range of pathways in the disease pathogenesis, from immune regulation to cholesterol biosynthesis. With increasing understanding of the basic biology underlying Rett syndrome, and improved understanding of the mouse models used for experimentation, the rapid growth of the field is only likely to increase in the coming years.

References

Abdala A, Bissonette J, Newman-Tancredi A (2014). Pinpointing brainstem mechanisms responsible for autonomic dysfunction in Rett syndrome: therapeutic perspectives for 5-HT1A agonists. *Front Physiol.* 5 (205); 1-8.

Abdala A, Dutschmann M, Bissonnette JM, Paton JF (2010). Correction of respiratory disorders in a mouse model of Rett syndrome. *PNAS U.S.A* 107(42); 18208-18213.

Ager S, Fyfe S, Christodoulou J, Jacoby P, Schmitt L, Leonard H (2006). Predictors of scoliosis in Rett syndrome. *J. Child Neurol.* 21; 809- 813.

Albright A, Gilmartin R, Swift D, Krach L, Ivanhoe C, McLaughlin J (2003). Long-term intrathecal baclofen therapy for sever spasticity of cerebral origin. *J. Neurosurg.* 98; 291-295.

Aman M, McDougle C, Scahill L, Handen B, Arnold L, Johnson C, Stigler K, Bearss K, Butter E, Swiezy N, Sukhodolsky D, Ramadan Y, Pozdol S, Nikolov R, Lecavalier L, Kohn A, Koenig K, Holloway J, Korzekwa P, Gavaletz A, Mulik J, Hall K, Dziura J, Ritz L, Trollinger S, Sunkyung Y, Vitiello B, Wagner A (2009). Medication and parent-training in children with pervasive developmental disorders and serious behaviour problems: results from a randomised-controlled trial. *Child Adolesc. Psych.* 48; 1143-1154.

Amir R, van der Veyver I, Wan M, Tran C, Franke U, Zoghbi H (1999). Rett syndrome is caused by mutations in X-linked MECP2, encoding methyl-CpG-binding protein 2. *Nat. Genet.* 23; 185-188.

Andaku D, Mercadante M, Schwartzman J (2005). Buspirone in Rett syndrome respiratory dysfunction. *Brain Dev.* 27; 437–438.

Armour A, Gottschlich M, Khoury J, Warden G, Kagan R (2008). A randomised controlled prospective trial of zolpidem and haloperidol for use as sleeping agents in paediatric burns patients. *J. Burn Care Res.* 29; 238-247.

Armstrong R, Steinbok P, Cochrane D, Kube S, Fife S, Farrell K, (1997). Intrathecally administered baclofen for treatment of children with spasticity of cerebral origin. *J. Neurosurg.* 87; 409-414.

Aron M (1990). The use and effectiveness of elbow splints in the Rett syndrome. *Brain Dev.* 12; 162-163.

Asaka Y, Jugloff D, Zhang L, Eubanks J, Fitsimonds R (2006). Hippocampal synaptic plasticity is impaired in the Mecp2-null mouse model of Rett syndrome. *Neurobiol. Dis.* 21; 217-227.

Assie M, Bardin L, Auclair A, Carilla-Durand E, Deeportiere R, Koek W, Kleven M, Colpaert F, Vacher B, Newmand-Tancredi A (2010). F15599, a highly selective post-synaptic 5-HT(1A) receptor agonist: in-vivo profile in behavioural models of antidepressant and serotonergic activity. *Int. J. Neuropsychopharmacol* 13(10):1285-98.

Badell, A (1991). The effect of medications that reduce spasticity in the management of spastic cerebral palsy. *J. Neurol. Rehabil* 5 (1 Suppl; 13–14

Baker S, Liptak G, Colletti R, Croffie J, Di Lorenzo C, Ector W, Nurko S (1999). Constipation in infants and children: evaluation and treatment. *J. Peadiatr Gastroenterol. Nutr.* 29(5); 612-626.

Ballas N, Lioy D, Grunseich C, Mandel G (2009). Non-cell autonomous influence of MeCP2-deficient glia on neuronal dendritic morphology. *Nat. Neurosci.* 12(3):311-7.

Ben-Zeev B, Aharoni R, Nissenkorn A, Arnon R (2011). Glatiramer acetate (GA, Copolymer-1) an hypothetical treatment option for Rett syndrome. *Med. Hypotheses* 76(2):190-3.

Blue M, Naidu S, Johnston M (1999). Development of amino acid receptors in frontal cortex from girls with Rett syndrome. *Ann. Neurol.* 45; 541-545.

Blumer J, Findling R, Shih W, Soubrane C, Reed M (2009). Controlled trial for zolpidem for the treatment of insomnia associated with attention-deficit/hyperactivity disorder in children 6 to 17 years of age. *Peaditarics* 123; e770-776.

Brendel C, Belakhov V, Werner H, Wegener E, Gartner J, Nudelman I, Baasov T, Huppke P (2011). Readthrough of nonsense mutations in Rett syndrome: evaluation of novel aminoglycosides and generation of a new mouse model. *J. Mol. Med.* 89; 398-398.

Brendel C, Klahold E, Gartner J, Huppke P (2009). Suppression of nonsense mutations in Rett syndrome by aminoglycoside antibiotics. *Paediatr. Res.* 65; 520-523.

Brucke T, Sofic E, Killian W, Rett A, Riederer P (1987). Reduced concentrations of and increased metabolism of biogenic amines in a single case of Rett syndrome; a post-mortem brain study. *J. Neural Transm.* 68; 315-324.

Buchovecky C, Turley S, Brown H, Kyle S, McDonald J, Liu B, Pieper A, Huang W, Katz D, Russell D, Shendure J, Justice M (2013). A suppressor screen in Mecp2 mutant mice implicates cholesterol metabolism in Rett syndrome. *Nat. Genet.* 45(9):1013-20.

Budden S (1997). Rett syndrome: habilitation and management reviewed. *Eur. Child Adol. Psych.* 1; 103-107.

Bumin G, Uyanik M, Yilmaz I, Kayihan H, Topcu M (2003). Hydrotherapy for Rett syndrome. *J. Rehabil. Med.* 35; 44-45.

Calfa G, Hablitz J, Pozzo-Miller (2011). Network hyperexcitability in hippocampal slices from MECP2 mutant mice revealed by voltage-sensitive dye imaging. *J. Neurophysiol.* 105; 1768-1784.

Carlson G (2012). Glutamate receptor dysfunction and drug targets across models of autism spectrum disorders. *Pharmacol. Biochem. Behav.* 100(4); 850-854.

Carnevali L, Mastorci F, Audero E, Graiani G, Rossi S, Macchi E, Callegari S, Bartolomucci A, Nalivaiko E, Quaini F, Gross C, Sgoifo A (2012). Stress-induced susceptibility to sudden cardiac death in mice with altered serotonin homeostasis. *PLoS One* 7(7):e41184.

Cassel S, Carouge D, Gensburger C, Anglard P, Burgun C, Dietrich JB, Aunis D, Zwiller J (2006). Fluoxetine and cocaine induce the epigenetic factors MeCP2 and MBD1 in adult rat brain. *Mol Pharmacol* 70(2):487-92.

Castro J, Garcia R, Kwok S, Banerjee A, Petravicz J, Woodson J, Mellios N, Tropea D, Sur M (2014). Functional recovery with recombinant human IGF-1 treatment in a mouse model of Rett syndrome. *Proc. Natl. Acad. Sci. U S A.* 111(27):9941-6.

Chahrour M, Zoghbi H (2007); The story of Rett syndrome: From clinic to neurobiology. *Neuron* 56; 422-437.

Chahrour M, Jung S, Shaw C, Zhou X,Wong S, Qin J, Zohgbi H (2008). MeCP2, a key contributor to neurological disease, activates and represses transcription. *Science* 320; 1224-1229.

Chang Q, Khare G, Dani V, Nelson S, Jaenisch R (2006). The disease progression of Mecp2 mutant mice is affected by the level of BDNF expression. *Neuron* 49(3); 341-348.

Chao H, Zoghbi H, Rosenmund R (2007). Mecp2 controls excitatory synaptic strength by regulating glutaminergic synapse number. *Neuron* 56; 58-65.

Chao H, Chen R, Samaco R, Xue M, Chahrour M, Yoo J, Neul J, Gong S, Lu H, Heintz N, Ekker M, Rubenstein J, Noebels J, Rosenmund C, Zoghbi H (2010). Dysfunction in GABA signalling mediates autism-like stereotypies and Rett syndrome phenotypes. *Nature* 468, 263–269.

Chapleau C, Lane J, Pozzo-Miller L, Percy A (2013). Evaluation of current pharmacological treatment options in the management of Rett syndrome: from present to future therapeutic alternatives. *Curr. Clin. Pharmacol.* 8(4); 358-369.

Chen R, Akbarian S, Tudor M, Jaenisch R (2001). Deficiency of methyl-CpG binding protein-2 in CNS neurons results in a Rett-like phenotype in mice. *Nat. Genet.* 27 327–331.

Chen Y, Hou L, Wang J (2008). HT1A/7 receptor agonist excites cardiac vagal neurons via inhibition of both GABAergic and glycinergic inputs. *Acta Pharmacol. Sin.* 29(5):529-38.

Chung CY, Chen CL, Wong A (2011). Pharmacotherapy of spasticity in children with cerebral palsy. *J. Formos Med. Assoc.* 110(4):215-22.

Christodoulou J, Grimm A, Maher T, Bennetts B (2003). RettBASE: The IRSA MECP2 variation database-a new mutation database in evolution. *Hum Mutat* 21; 466–472.

Corvin A, Molinos I, Little G, Donohoe G, Gill M, Morris D, Tropea D (2012). Insulin-like growth factor (IGF-1) and its active peptide (1-3)IGF1 enhance the expression of synaptic markers in neuronal circuits through different cellular machanisms. *Neurosci. Lett.* 520(1):51-6.

Dahlin M, Knutsson E, Nergardh A (1993). Treatment of spasticity in children with low-dose benzodiazepines. *J Neurol Sci* 177; 54-60.

Dai A, Wasay M, Awan S (2008). Botulinum toxin type A with oral baclofen versus oral tizanidine: a nonrandomized pilot comparison in patients with cerebral palsy and spastic equinus foot deformity. *J. Child Neurol.* 23(12):1464-6.

Dan B, Motta F, Vles J, Vloeberghs M, Becher J, Euson P, Gautheron V, Lutjen S, Mall V, Pascual-Pascual S, Pauwels P, Roste G (2010). Consensus on the appropriate use of intrathecal baclofen therapy in paediatric spasticity. *Euro J. Paediatr. Neurol.* 14; 19-28.

Dani V, Chang Q, Maffei A, Turrigiano G, Jaenisch R, Nelson S (2005). Reduced cortical activity due to a shift in the balance between excitation and inhibition in a mouse model of Rett syndrome. *PNAS* 102; 12560-12565.

Dani V, Nelson S (2009). Intact long-term potentiation but reduced connectivity between neocortical layer 5 pyramidal neurons in a mouse model of Rett syndrome. *J. Neurosci.* 29; 11263-11270.

De Felice C, Signorini C, Durand T, Ciccoli L , Leoncini S, D'Esposito M, Filosa S, Oger C, Guy A, Bultel-Ponce V, Galano J, Pecorelli A, De Felice L, Valacchi G, Hayek J (2012). Partial rescue of Rett syndrome by ω-3 polyunsaturated fatty acids (PUFAs) oil. *Genes Nutr.* 7; 447-458.

De Felice C, Signorini C, Leoncini S, Pecorelli A, Durand T, Valacchi G, Ciccoli L, Hayek J (2012). The role of oxidative stress in Rett syndrome: an overview. *Ann. NY Acad. Sci.* 1259; 121-135.

De Felice C, Della Ragione F, Signorini C, Leoncini S, Pecorelli A, Ciccoli L, Scalabrì F, Marracino F, Madonna M, Belmonte G, Ricceri L, De Filippis B, Laviola G, Valacchi G, Durand T, Galano JM, Oger C, Guy A, Bultel-Poncé V, Guy J, Filosa S, Hayek J, D'Esposito M (2014). Oxidative brain damage in Mecp2-mutant murine models of Rett syndrome. *Neurobiol. Dis.*. 68: 66-77.

Deogracias R, Yazdani M, Dekkers MP, Guy J, Ionescu MC, Vogt KE, Barde YA (2012). Fingolimod, a sphingosine-1 phosphate receptor modulator, increases BDNF levels and improves symptoms of a mouse model of Rett syndrome. *Proc. Natl. Acad. Sci. U S A* 109(35): 14230-14235.

Depoortère R, Auclair AL, Bardin L, Colpaert FC, Vacher B, Newman-Tancredi A (2010). F15599, a preferential post-synaptic 5-HT1A receptor agonist: activity in models of cognition in comparison with reference 5-HT1A receptor agonists. *Eur. Neuropsychopharmacol.* 20(9):641-54.

D'Ercole A, Ye P, Calikoglu A, Gutierrez-Ospina G (1996). The role of insulin-like growth factors in the central nervous system. *Mol. Neurobiol.* 13; 227-255.

Derecki N, Cronk J, Lu Z, Xu E, Abbott S, Guyenet P, Kipnis J (2012). Wild-type microglia arrest pathology in a mouse model of Rett syndrome. *Nature* 484; 105-109.

Derecki N, Cronk J, Kipnis J (2013). The role of microglia in brain maintenance: implications for Rett syndrome. *Trends Immunol.* 34(3); 144-150.

Donovan W, Carter R, Rossi C, Wilkerson M (1988). Clonidine effect on spasticity: a clinical trial. *Arch. Physic. Med. Rehab.* 69; 193-194.

Dressler A, Stocklin B, Reithofer E, Benninger F, Freilinger M, Hauser E, Reiter-Fink E, Seidl R, Trimmel-Schwahofer P, Feucht M (2010). Long-term outcome and tolerability of the ketogenic diet in drug-resistant childhood epilepsy. *Seizure* 19; 404-408.

El-Khoury R, Panayotis N, Matagne V, Ghata A, Villard L, Roux JC (2014). GABA and glutamate pathways are spatially and developmentally affected in the brain of Mecp2-deficient mice. *PLoS One* 9(3); e92169.

Ellaway C, Williams K, Leonard H, Higgins G, Christodoulou J (1999). Rett syndrome: randomised-controlled trial of L-carnitine. *J. Child Neurol.* 14; 162-167.

Ellaway C, Peat J, Williams K, Leonard H, Christodoulou (2001A). Medium-term open-label trial of L-carnitine in Rett syndrome. *Brain and Devel* 23(1); S81-S89.

Ellaway C, Christodoulou J (2001B). Rett syndrome: clinical characteristics and recent genetic advances. *Disabil Rehabil* 23; 98-106.

Emslie G, Heiligenstein J, Wagner K, Hoog S, Ernest D, Nilsson M, Jacobson J (2002). Fluoexetine for acute treatment of depression in children and adolescents: a placebo-controlled, randomised clinical trial. *Child Adolesc. Psych.* 41; 1205-1215.

Enns G, Kinsman S, Perlman S, Spicer K, Abdenur J, Cohen B, Amagata A, Barnes A, Kheifets V, Shrader W, Thoolen M, Blankenburg F, Miller G (2012). Initial experience in the treatment of inherited mitochondrial disease with EPI-743. *Mol Genet Metab* 105; 91-102.

Erman M, Seiden D, Zammit G, Sainati S, Zhang J (2006). An efficacy, safety and dose-response study of Ramelton in patients with chronic primary insomnia. *Sleep Med.* 7; 17-24.

Felt B, Wise C, Olson A, Kochhar P, Marcus S, Coran A (1999). Guideline for management of paediatric idiopathic constipation and soiling. *Arch. Pediatr Adolesc. Med.* 153(4):380-385.

Fitzgerald P, Jankovic J, Percy A (1990). Rett syndrome and associated movement disorders. *Movement Disorders* 5(3); 195-202.

Fox (1992). A critical period for experience-dependent synaptic plasticity in rat barrel cortex. *J. Neurosci.* 12; 1826-1838.

France K, Blampied M, Wilkinson P (1991). Treatment of infant sleep disturbance by trimeprazine in combination with extinction. *Journal of Developmental and Behavioural Paediatrics* 12; 308-314.

Freilinger M, Dunkler D, Lanator I, Item CB, Mühl A, Fowler B, Bodamer OA (2011). Effects of creatine supplementation in Rett syndrome: a randomized, placebo-controlled trial. *J. Dev. Behav. Pediatr.* 32(6):454-60

Gardalla K, Bailey M, Stuart S (2011). MeCP2 and Rett syndrome: reversibility and potential avenues for therapy. *Biochem. J.* 439; 1-14.

Garg S, Lioy D, Cheval H, McGann J, Bissonette J, Murtha M, Foust K, Kaspar B, Bird A, Mandel G (2013). Systemic delivery of MeCP2 rescues behavioural and cellular deficits in female mouse models of Rett syndrome. *J. Neurosci.* 33; 13612-13620.

Gerszten P, Albright A, Johnstone G (1998). Intrathecal baclofen infusion and subsequent orthopedic surgery in patients with spastic cerebral palsy. *J. Neurosurg.* 88; 1009–1013.

Giacometti E, Luikenhuis S, Beard C, Jaenisch R (2007). Partial rescue of MeCP2 deficiency by postnatal activation of MeCP2 *Proc. Natl. Acad. Sci. USA* 104; 1931–1936.

Gionnotti F, Cortesi F, Cerquiglini A, Bernabei P (2006). An open-label study of controlled release melatonin in treatment of sleep disorders in children with autism. *J. Autism Dev. Disord.* 36: 741-752.

Glaze D, Frost J, Schultz et al., (1989). Effect of naloxone on breathing, hand movements, electroencephalogram during wakefulness in patients with rett syndrome. *Ann. Neurol.* 26; 486.

Glaze D, Schultze R, Frost D (1998). Rett syndrome: Characterisation of seizures versus non-seizures. *Electroencephalo Clin. Neurophysiol.* 106; 78-83.

Glaze D, Percy A, Motil K, Lane J, Isaacs J, Schultz R, Barrish J, Neul J, O'Brian W, Smith E (2009). A study of the treatment of Rett syndrome with folate and betaine. *J. Child Neurol.* 24(5); 551-556.

Glaze D, Percy A, Skinner S, Motil K, Neul J, Barrish J, Lane J, Geerts S, Annese F, Graham R, McNair S, Lee H (2010). Epilepsy and the natural history of Rett syndrome. *Neurology* 74(11) 909-912.

Gokben S, Ardik U, Serdaroglu G (2012). Use of buspirone and fluoxetine for breathing problems in Rett syndrome. *Paediatr Neurol* 46(3); 192-194.

Gorbachevskaya N, Bashina V, Gratchev V, Iznak A (2001). Cerebrolysin therapy in Rett syndrome: clinical and EEG mapping study. *Brain Dev.* 2001 Dec;23 Suppl 1:S90-3.

Gross C, Zhuang X, Stark K, Ramboz S, Oosting R, Kirby L, Santarelli L, Beck S, Hen R (2002). Serotonin1A receptor acts during development to establish normal anxiety-like behaviour in the adult. *Nature* 416(6879):396-400.

Guideri F, Acampa M, Blardi P, de Lalla A, Zappella M, Hayek Y (2004). Cardiac dysautonomia and serotonin plasma levels in Rett syndrome. *Neuropediatrics* 35(1):36-8.

Guideri F, Acampa M, Hayek Y, Zapella M (2005). Effects of acetyl-L-carnitine on cardiac dysautonomia in Rett syndrome: Prevention of sudden death? *Paediatr Cardiol* 26; 574-577.

Guy J, Hendrich B, Holmes M, Martin J, Bird A (2001). A mouse Mecp2-null mutation causes neurological symptoms that mimic Rett syndrome. *Nat. Genet.* 27 322–326.

Guy J, Gan J, Selfridge S, Cobb S, Bird A (2007). Reversal of neurological defects in a mouse model of Rett syndrome. *Science* 315; 1143-1147.

Haas R, Rice M, Trauner D, Merritt T, Opitz J (1986). Therapeutic effects of a ketogenic diet in Rett syndrome. *Amer. J. Med. Gen. Suppl.* 1; 225-246.

Hagberg B, Witt-Engerstrom I (1986). Rett syndrome; a suggested staging system for describing impairment profile with increasing age towards adolescence. *Amer. J. Med. Genet.* 24; 47-59.

Hagberg B, Anvret M, Wahlstrom J (1993). Rett syndrome: clinical and biological aspects. MacKeith Press London.

Hagebeuk EE, Koelman JH, Duran M, Abeling NG, Vyth A, Poll-The BT (2011). Clinical and electroencephalographic effects of folinic acid treatment in Rett syndrome patients. *Child Neurol.* 26(6):718-23.

Hagebeuk EE, Duran M, Koelman JH, Abeling NG, Vyth A, Poll-The BT (2012). Folinic acid supplementation in Rett syndrome patients does not influence the course of the disease: a randomized study. *J. Child Neurol.* 27(3):304-9.

Hamberger A, Gillberg C, Palm A, Hagberg B (1992). Elevated CSF glutamate in Rett syndrome. *Neuropaediatr* 23; 212-213.

Hampson D, Gholizadeh S, Pacey L (2012). Pathways to drug development for autisdm spectrum disorders. *Clin. Pharmacol. Ther.* 91; 189-200.

Hanks S (1990). Motor disabilities in Rett syndrome and physical therapy strategies. *Brain and Development* 12(1); 157-161.

Hennessy H, Chez M (2009). Pediatric safety of tizanidine: clinical adverse event database and retrospective chart assessment. *Paediatr Drugs* 11(6):397-406.

Holloway J, Aman M (2011). Pharmacological treatment of sleep disturbance in developmental disabilities: a review of the literature. *Res. Dev. Disabil* 32; 939-962.

Hoving M, van Raak E, Spincemaille G, Palmans L, Becher J, Vles J (2009). Efficacy of intrathecal baclofen therapy in children with intractable spastic cerebral palsy: a randomised controlled trial. *Eur. J. Paediatr Neuro.* 13(3):240-6.

Huppke P, Kohler K, Brockmann K, Stettner G, Gartner J (2007). Treatment of epilepsy in Rett syndrome. *Euro J. Paediatr. Neurol.* 11; 10-16.

Ide S, Itoh M, Goto Y (2005). Defect in normal developmental increase in the brain biogenic amine concentrations in the mecp2-null mouse. *Neurosci. Lett.* 386(1); 14-17.

Ingrassia A, Turk J (2005). The use of clonidine for severe and intractable sleep problems in children with neurodevelopmental disorders: A case series. *Euro Child Adolesc. Psych.* 14; 34-40.

Jian L, Nagarajan L, de Klerk N, Ravine D, Christodoulou J, Leonard H (2007). Seizures in Rett syndrome: An overview from a one-year calendar study. *Euro J. Paediatr. Neurol.* 11; 310-317.

Johnston M, Jeon O, Pevsner J, Blue M, Naidu S (2001). Neurobiology of Rett syndrome: a genetic disorder of synapse development. *Brain Dev.* 23; S206-S213.

Johnson R, Lam M, Punzo A, Li H, Lin B, Ye K, Mitchell G, Chang Q, (2012). 7,8-dihydroxyflavone exhibits therapeutic efficacy in a mouse model of Rett syndrome. *J. Appl. Psychol.* 112(5); 704-710.

Julu PO, Kerr AM, Hansen S, Apartopoulos F, Jamal GA. Immaturity of medullary cardiorespiratory neurones leading to inappropriate autonomic reactions as a likely cause of sudden death in Rett's syndrome (1997). *Arch. Dis. Child* 77:464-5.

Julu P, Kerr A, Apartopoulos F, Al-Rawas SEngerstrom I, Engerstrom L, Jamal G, Hansen S (2001). Characterisation of breathing and associated autonomic dysfunction in the Rett disorder. *Arch. Dis. Child* 85; 29-37.

Julu P, Engerstrom I, Hansen S, Apartopopulos F, Engerstrom B, Pini G, Delamont R, Smeets E (2008). Addressing the cardiorespiratory challenges posed by Rett syndrome in Medicine; The Froso Declaration. *Lancet* 371; 1981-1983.

Kadyan V, Clairmont A, Goerge R, Johnson E (2003). Intrathecal baclofen for spasticity management in Rett syndrome. *Am. J. Phys. Me. Rehabil* 82: 560–562.

Kalia L, Kalia S, Salter M (2008). NMDA receptors in clinical neurology: excitatory times ahead. *Lancet Neurol.* 7; 742-755.

Katz D, Berger-Sweeney J, Eubanks J, Justice M, Neul J, Pozzo-Miller L, Blue M, Christian D, Crawley J, Guistetto M, Guy J, Howell J, Kron M, Nelson S, Samaco R, Schaevitz L, Hillaire-Clarke C, Young J, Zoghbi H, Mamounas L (2012). Preclinicla research in Rett syndrome: setting the foundation for translational success. *Dis. Mod. Mech.* 5; 733-745.

Keane D (2006). A systematic review of the use of the ketogenic diet in childhood epilepsy. *Paediatr Neurol* 35; 1-5.

Kerr AM, Armstrong DD, Prescott RJ, Doyle D, Kearney DL. Rett syndrome: analysis of deaths in the British survey (1997). *Eur. Child Adolesc. Psych.*;6 Suppl 1:71-4.

Kerr A, Julu P (1999). Recent insights into hyperventilation from the study of Rett syndrome. Arch Dis Child 80; 384-387.

Kerr A, Webb P, Prescott R, Milne Y (2003). Results of surgery for scoliosis in Rett syndrome. *J. Child Neurol.*; 18: 703-708.

King B, Hollander E, Sikich L, McCracken J, Scahill L, Bregman J, Donnelly C, Anagnostou E, Sullivan L, Hirtz D, Wagner A Ritz L (2009). Lack of efficacy of citalopram in children with autism spectrum disorders and high levels of repetitive behaviour. *Arch. Gen. Psych.* 66; 583-590.

Kline D, Ogier M, Kunze D, Katz D (2010). Exogenous brain-derived neurotrophic factor rescues synaptic dysfunction in Mecp2 null mice. *J. Neurosci.* 30; 5303–5310.

Koman L, Mooney J, Smith B, Walker F, Leon J, the BOTOX study group (2000). Botulinum toxin type A neuromuscular blockade in the treatment of lower extremity spasticity in cerebral palsy: a randomised, double-blind, placebo-controlled trial. *J. Paediatr Orthop.* 20; 108- 115.

Kondo M, Gray L, Pelka G, Christodoulou J, Tam P, Hannan A (2008). Environmental enrichment ameliorates a motor coordination deficit in a mouse model of Rett syndrome--Mecp2 gene dosage effects and BDNF expression. *Eur. J. Neurosci.* 27(12):3342-50.

Krach L (2001). Pharmacotherapy of spasticity: Oral medications and intrathecal baclofen. *J. Child Neurol.* 16; 31-36.

Lally P, Bischoff A, Richter D (1994). Seritonin 1A receptor activation suppresses respiratory apneusis in the cat. *Neurosci. Let.* 172; 59-62.

Lappalainen R, Riikonen R (1996). High levels of cerebrospinal fluid glutamate in Rett syndrome. *Paediatr. Neurol.* 15; 213-216.

Larsson G, Engerstrom I (2001). Gross motor ability in Rett syndrome- the power of expectation, motivation and planning. *Brain and Development* 23; S77-S81.

LaSalle J, Goldstine J, Balmer D, Greco C (2001). Quantitative localisation of heterogeneous methyl-CpG-binding protein 2 (MeCP2) expression phenotypes in normal and Rett syndrome brain by laser scanning cytometry. *Hum. Mol. Genet.* 10; 1729-1740.

Lee J, Lee K, Lee Y, Choi Y, Park C, Park S, Jung D, Lee C (2013). Botulinum Toxin Treatment on Upper Limb Function in School Age Children With Bilateral Spastic Cerebral Palsy: One Year Follow-up. *Ann. Rehabil. Med.* 37(3):328-35

Leibhaber G, Riemann E, Baumeister F (2003). Ketogenic diet in Rett syndrome. *J. Child Neurol.* 18; 74-75.

Lekman A, Witt-Engerstrom I, Gottfries J, Hagberg A, Percy A (1989). Rett syndrome; biogenic amines and metabolites in post-mortem brain. *Paediatr. Neurol.* 5; 357-362.

Leonardo E, Hen R (2008). Anxiety as a developmental disorder. *Neuropsychopharmacology* 33(1):134-40.

Levitt E , Hunnicutt B, Knopp S, Williams J, Bissonnette J (2013). A selective 5HT1A receptor agonist improves respiration in a mouse model of Rett syndrome. *J. Appl. Psychol.* 115; 1626-1633.

Li W, Pozzo-Miller (2014). BDNF deregulation in Rett syndrome. *Neuropharmacol* 76; 737-746.

Lidstrom J, Stokland E, Hagberg B (1994). Scoliosis in Rett syndrome: clinical and biological aspects. *Spine* 19(14);

Lioy D, Garg S, Monaghan C, Raber J, Foust K, Kaspar B, Hirrlinger P, Kirchhoff F, Bissonnette J, Ballas N, Gail M (2011). A role for glia in the progression of Rett's syndrome. *Nature* 475; 497-500.

Lonetti G, Angelucci A, Morando L, Boggio E, Guisetto M, Pizzorusso T (2010). Early environmental enrichment moderates the behavioural and synaptic phenotype in Mecp2 null mice. *Biol. Psych.* 67; 657-665.

Lotan M, Isakov E, Merrick J (2004). Improving functional skills and physical fitness in children with Rett syndrome. *J. Intell Disabil Res.* 48; 730-735.

Loton M, Zysman L (2006). The digestive system and nutritional considerations for individuals with Rett syndrome. *TheScientificWorld Journal* 6; 1737-1749.

Lubshc L, Habersang R, Haase M, Luedtke S (2006). Oral baclofen and clonidine for treatment of spasticity in children. *J. Child Neurol.* 21; 1090-1092.

Luikenhuis S, Giacometti E, Beard C, Jaenisch R (2004). Expression of MeCP2 in post-mitotic neurons rescues Rett syndrome in mice. *PNAS* 101; 6033-6038.

Lynn A, Turner M, Chambers H (2009). Surgical management of spasticity in persons with cerebral palsy. *PM&R* 1; 834-838.

Maezawa I, Jin L. (2010). Rett syndrome microglia damage dendrites and synapses by the elevated release of glutamate. *J. Neurosci.* 30(15): 5346-56.

Marchand V, Motil K, NASPGHAN Committee on Nutrition (2006). Nutrition support for neurologically impaired children: A clinical report of the

North American Socfiety for Paediatric Gastroenterology, Hepatology and Nutrition. *J. Paediatr Gastroenterol. Nutr.* 43; 123-135.

Marcus R, Owen R, Kamen L, Manos G, McQuade R, Carson W, Aman M (2009). A placebo-controlled, fixed dose study of aripiprazole in children and adolescents with irritability associated with autistic disorder. *Child Adolesc. Psych.* 48; 1110-1119.

Mathur S, Chu S, McCormick Z, Chang Chien G, Marciniak C. (2014) Long-term Intrathecal Baclofen: Outcomes After More than 10 Years of Treatment. *PM&R* 6:6, 506-513.e1.

McArthur A, Budden S (1998). Sleep dysfunction in Rett syndrome: A trial of exogenous melatonin treatment. *Developmental Medicine and Child Neurology* 40; 186-192.

McCauley M, Wang T, Mike E, Herrera J, Beavers D, Huang TW, Ward C, Skinner S, Percy A, Glaze D, Wehrens X, Neul J (2011). Pathogenesis of Lethal Cardiac Arrhythmias in Mecp2 Mutant Mice: Implication for Therapy in Rett Syndrome. *Sci. Transl. Med.* 3; Article ID 113ra125.

Medrihan L, Tantalaki E, Aramuni G, Sargsyan V, Dudanova I, Missler M, Zhang W (2008). Early defects of GABAergic synapses in the brainstem of a MeCP2 mouse model of Rett syndrome. *J. Neurophysiol.* 99; 112-121.

Meins M, Lehman J, Garresheim F, Herchenbach J, Hagedorn M, Hameister K, Epplen J (2005). Submicroscopic duplication in Xq28 causes increased expression of the MECP2 gene in a boy with severe mental retardation and features of Rett syndrome. *J. Med. Genet.* 42 e12.

Merenstein D, Diener-West M, Halbower A, Krist A, Rubin H (2006). The trial of infant response to diphenhydramine: The TIRED study. *Arch. Paed Adolesc. Med.* 150; 707-712.

Milla P, Jackson A (1977). A controlled trial of baclofen in children with cerebral palsy. *J. Int. Med. Res.* 5(6):398-404.

Ming X, Gordon E, Kang N, Wagner G (2008). Use of clonidine with autism spectrum disorders. *Brain Dev.* 30; 454-460.

Miyamoto A, Oki J, Takahashi S, Okuno A (1999). Serum melatonin kinetics and long-term melatonin treatment for sleep disorders in Rett syndrome. *Brain and Development* 21(1); 59-62.

Mohandas T, Sparkes R, Shapiro L (1981). Reactivation of an inactive human X chromosome: evidence for X inactivation by DNA methylation. *Science* 211; 393-396.

Molenaers G, Fagard K, Van Campenhout A, Desloovere K (2013). Botulinum toxin A treatment of the lower extremities in children with cerebral palsy. *J. Child Orthop* 7(5):383-7.

Morretti P, Levenson J, Battaglia F, Atkinson R, Teague R, Antalffy B, Armstrong D, Arancio O, Sweatt D Zoghbi H (2006). Learning and Memory and Synaptic Plasticity Are Impaired in a Mouse Model of Rett Syndrome. *J. Neurosci.* 26; 319-327.

Motil K, Schultz R, Brown B, Glaze D, Percy A (1994). Altered energy balance may account for growth failure in Rett syndrome. *J. Child Neurol.* 9(3); 315-319.

Motil K, Ellis K, Barrish J, Caeg E, Glaze D (2008). Bone mineral content and bone mineral density are lower in older than in younger females with Rett syndrome. *Peadiatr Res.* 64; 435-439.

Motil K, Morrissey M, Caeg E, Barrish J, Glaze D (2009). Gastrostomy placement improves height and weight gain in girls with Rett syndrome. *J. Paediatr. Gastroenterol. Nutr.* 49(2); 237-242.

Motil K, Caeg E, Barrish J, Geerts S Lane J, Percy A, Annese F, McNair L, Skinner S, Lee H, Neul J, Glaze D (2012). Gastrointestinal and nutritional problems occur frequently throughout life in girls and women with Rett syndrome. *J. Paediatr. Gastroenterol. Nutr.* 55(3); 292-298.

Motta F, Antonello C (2014). Analysis of complications in 430 consecutive pediatric patients treated with intrathecal baclofen therapy: 14-year experience. *J. Neurosurg. Pediatr* 13(3):301-6.

Nag N, Berger-Sweeney J (2007). Post-natal dietary choline supplementation alters behavior in a mouse model of Rett syndrome. *Neurobiol. Dis.*. 26; 473-480.

Nag N, Mellott T, Berger-Sweeney J (2008). Effects of postnatal dietary choline supplementation on motor regional brain volume and growth factor expression in a mouse model of Rett syndrome. *Brain Res.* 1237; 101-109.

Nag N, Moriuchi J, Peitzman C, Ward B, Kolodny N, Berger-Sweeney J (2009). Environmental enrichment alters locomotor behaviour and ventricular volume in Mecp2 1lox mice. *Behav. Brain Res.* 196; 44-48.

Naganuma G, Bellingsley F (1988). Effects of hand splints on stereotypic hand behaviour of three girls with Rett syndrome. *Phys. Ther* 68; 664-671.

Naidu S, Kaufmann W, Abrams M, Pearlman G, Lanham D, Frederickson K, Barker P, Horska A, Golay X, Mori S, Wong D, Yablonski M, Moser H, Johnston M (2001). Neuroimaging studies in Rett syndrome. *Brain Dev.* 23; S62-S71.

Nakamura K, Koyama Y, Takahashi K, Tsurui H, Xui Y, Ohtsuji M et al., (2006). Requirement of tryptophan hydroxylase during development for maturation of sensorimotor gating. *J. Mol. Biol.* 363; 345-354.

Namerow L, Prakesh T, Bostic J, Prince J, Monuteaux M (2003). Use of Citalopram in Pervasive Developmental Disorders. *J. Dev. Behav. Paediatr* 24; 104-108.

Nan X, Campoy F, Bird A (1997). MeCP2 is a transcriptional repressor with abundant binding sites in genomic chromatin. *Cell* 88; 471-481.

Neal E, Chaffe H, Schwartz R, Lawson M, Edwards N, Fitzsimmons G, Whitney A, Cross J (2008). The ketogenic diet for the treatment of childhood epilepsy: a randomised controlled trial. *Lancet Neurol* 7; 500-506.

Newman-Tancredi A, Martel J, Assié M, Buritova J, Lauressergues E, Cosi C, Heusler P, Bruins Slot L, Colpaert F, Vacher B, Cussac D (2009). Signal transduction and functional selectivity of F15599, a preferential post-synaptic 5-HT1A receptor agonist. *Br. J. Pharmacol.* 156(2):338-353.

Nikitina T, Shi X, Ghosh R, Horowitz-Scherer R, Hansen J Woodcock C (2007A). Multiple modes of interaction between the methylated DNA-binding protein MeCP2 and chromatin. *Mol. Cell Biol.* 27; 864-877.

Nikitina T, Ghosh R, Horowitz-Scherer R, Hansen J, Grigoryev S, Woodcock C (2007B). MeCP2-Chromatin Interactions Include the Formation of Chromatosome-like Structures and Are Altered in Mutations Causing Rett Syndrome. *J. Biol. Chem.* 282; 28237-28245.

Nissencorn A, Gak E, Vecsler M, Reznik H, Menascu S, Zeev B (2010). Epilepsy in Rett syndrome- the experience of the national Rett centre. *Epilepsia* 51(7); 1252-1258.

Nudelman I, Rebibo-Sabbah A, Cherniavsky M, Belakhov V, Hainrichson M, Chen F, Schacht J, Pilch D, Ben-Yosef T, Baasov T (2009). Development of novel aminoglycoside (NB54) with reduced toxicity and enhanced suppression of disease-causing mutations. *J. Med. Chem* 52; 2836-2845.

Ogier M, Wang H, Hong E, Wang Q, Greenberg M, Katz D (2007). Brain-derived neurotrophic factor expression and respiratory function improve after ampakine treatment in a mouse model of Rett syndrome. *J. Neurosci.* 27(40); 10912-10917.

Okabe Y, Takahashi T, Mitsumasu C, Kosai K, Tanaka E, Matsuishi T (2012). Alterations of gene expression and glutamate clearance in astrocytes derived from a MECP2-null mouse model of Rett syndrome. *PLoS One* 7; e35354.

Ormazabal A, Artuch R, Vilaseca MA, Aracil A, Pineda M (2005). Cerebrospinal fluid concentrations of folate, biogenic amines and pterins in Rett syndrome: treatment with folinic acid. *Neuropediatrics.* 36(6):380-5.

Ottaviano S, Gianotti F, Cortesi F (1991). The effect of niaprazine on some common sleep disorders in children; a double-blind clinical trial by means of continuos home-video recorded sleep. *Child's Nervous System* 7; 332-335.

Owen R, Sikich L, Marcus R, Corey-Lisle P, Manos G, McQuade R, Carson W, Findling R (2009). Aripiprazole in the treatment of irritability in children and adults with autistic disorder. *Am. Aca.d Paediatrics* 124; 1533-1540.

Pan CH, Tsai SJ (2011). Early intervention with psychostimulants or antidepressants to increase methyl-CpG-binding protein 2 (MeCP2) expressions: A potential therapy for Rett syndrome. *Med. Sci. Monit.* 18(1): HY1-3

Paul I, Yoder K, Crowell K, Shaffer M, McMillan H, Carlson L et al., (2004). Effect of dextromethorphan, diohenhydramine, and placebo on nocturnal cough and sleep quality for coughing children and their parents. *Paediatrics* 114; e85-e90.

Percy A, Glaze D, Schultz R, Zoghbi H, Williamson D, Frost J, Jankovic J, del Junco D, Skender M, Waring S, Myer E (1994). Rett syndrome: Controlled study of an oral opiate antagonist, naltrexone. *Ann. Neurol.* 35; 464-470.

Percy A (2002). Clinical trials and treatment prospects. *Mental Retard Dev. Disabil Res. Rev.* 8; 106-111.

Percy A, Lane J (2005). Rett syndrome: Model of neurodevelopmental disorders. *J. Child Neurol.* 20; 718- 721.

Percy A (2014). Rett syndrome: Coming to terms with treatment. *Advances Neurosci* Article ID 345270.

Phillips L, Appleton R, (2004). Systematic review of melatonin treatment in children with neurodevelopmental disabilities and sleep impairment. *Developmental Medicine and Child Neurology* 46; 771-775

Pini G, Scusa M, Felloni B, Congiu L, Benincasa A, Frati R, Bottiglioni I, Di Marco P, Borelli P, Bonuccelli U, Della-Chiesa A, Prina-Mello A, Tropea D (2012). Safety assessment of IGF-1 treatment: study on six Rett patients. *Autism Res. Treatm* 679801, Epub Jun 13.

Pini G, Scusa M, Benincasa A, Bottiglioni I, Congiu L, Vadhatpour C, Romanelli A, Gemo I, Puccetti C, McNamara R, O'Leary S, Corvin A,

Gill M, Tropea D (2014). Repeated insulin-like growth factor-1 treatment in a patient with Ret syndrome: a single case study. *Front Paediatr* 2; 1-10.

Pintaudi M, Grazia Calevo M, Vignoli A, Parodi E, Aiello F, Baglietto M, Hayek Y, Buoni S, Renieri A, Russo S, Cogliati F, Giordano L, Canaveni M, Veneselli E (2010). Epilepsy in Rett syndrome: Clinical and genetic features. *Epilepsy & Behaviour* 19; 296-300.

Plioplys A, Kasnicka I (1993). L-carnitine as a treatment for Rett syndrome. *Southern Med. J.* 86; 1411-1412.

Plochl E, Sperl W, Wermuth B, Colombo J (1996). Carnitine deficiency and carnitine therapy in a patient with Rett syndrome. *Klin. Paediatr* 208; 129-134.

Posey D, Guenn K, Kohn A, Swiezy N, McDougle C (2001). A naturalistic open-label study of mirtazapine in autistic and other pervasive developmental disorders. *J. Child Adolesc. Psychopharmacol* 11; 267-277.

Popescu A, Sidorova E, Zhang G, Eubanks J (2010). Aminoglycoside-mediated patiral suppression of MECP2 nonsense mutations responsible for Rett syndrome in vitro. *J. Neurosci. Res* 88; 2316-2324.

Pranzatelli M, Tate E, Dukart W, Flint M, Hoffman M, Oksa A (2005). Sleep disturbance and rage attacks in opsoclonus-myoclonus syndrome: response to trazodone. *J. Paediatr* 147; 372-378.

Richardson G (2004). Serotonergic neurons as carbon dioxide sensors that maintain pH homeostasis. *Nat Rev Neurosci* 5(6); 449-461

Rossi P, Posar A, Parmeggiani A (1999). Niaprazine in the treatment of autistic disorder. *J. Child Neurol.* 14; 547-550.

Roth T, Seiden D, Sainati S, Wang-Weigand S, Zhang J, Zee P (2006). Effects of Ramelton on patient-reported sleep latency in older adults with chronic insomnia. *Sleep Med.* 7; 312-318.

Roux JC, Dura E, Moncla A, Mancini J, Villard L (2007). Treatment with desipramine improves breathing and survival in a mouse model for Rett syndrome *Euro J. Neurosci.* 25; 1915-1922.

Roux JC, Dura E, Villard L (2008). Tyrosine hydroxylase deficit in the chemoafferent and the sympathoadrenergic pathways of the Mecp2-deficient mouse. *Neurosci. Lett.* 447; 82-86.

Roux JC, Panayotis N, Dyra E, Villard L (2010). Progressive noradrenergic deficits in the locus ceruleus of Mecp2 deficient mice. *J. Neurosci. Res.* 88; 1500-1509.

Russell J, Blue M, Johnston M, Naidu S, Hossain M (2007). Enhanced cell death in MeCP2 null cerebellar granule neurons exposed to excitotoxicity and hypoxia. *Neuroscience* 150; 563–574.

Russo R, Vymutt J, Gurura J, Allen J (1976). The effectiveness of diphenhydramine in paediatric sleep disorders. *J. Clin. Pharmacol.* 284-288.

Samaco R, Mendel-Brehm C, Chao HT, Ward C, Fyffe-Maricich S, Ren J, Hyland K, Thaller C, Maricich S, Humphreys P, Greer J, Percy A, Glaze D, Zoghbi H, Neul J (2008). Loss of MECP2 in aminergic neurons causes cell-autonomous defects in neurotransmitter synthesis and specific behavioural abnormalities. *PNAS U.S.A* 106(51); 21966-21971.

Sansom D, Krishnan V, Corbett J, Kerr A (1993). Emotional and behavioural aspects of Rett syndrome. *Dev. Med. Child Neurol.* 35(4); 340-345.

Sampson F, Hayward A Evans G, Morton R, Collette B (2002). Functional benefits and cost-benefit analysis of continuous intrathecal baclofen infuction for management of severe spasticity. *J. Neurosurg.* 96; 1052-1057.

Scheinberg A, Hall K, Lam LT, O'Flaherty S (2006) Oral baclofen in children with cerebral palsy: a double-blind cross-over pilot study. *J. Paediatr Child Health* 42(11):715-20.

Schmid D, Yang T, Ogier M, Adams I, Mirakhur Y, Wang Q, Massa S, Longo F, Katz D (2012). A TrkB small molecule partial agonist rescues TrkB phosphorylation deficits and improves respiratory function in a mouse model of Rett syndrome. *J. Neurosci.* 32(5); 1803-1810.

Schultz R, Glaze D, Motil K, Herbert D Percy A (1988). Hand and foot growth failure in Rett syndrome. *J. Child Neurol.* 13(2); 71-74.

Schultz R, Glaze D, Motil K, Armstrong D, del Junco D, Hubbard C, Percy A (1993). The pattern of growth failure in Rett syndrome. *Am. J. Dis. Child.* 147:633-7.

Sees J, Miller F (2013). Overview of foot deformity management in children with cerebral palsy. *J. Child Orthop* 7(5):373-7.

Shahbazian M, Antaffy B, Armstron G, Zoghbi H (2002). Insight into Rett syndrome: MeCP2 levels display tissue- and cell-specific differences and correlate with neuronal maturation. *Hum. Mol. Genet* 11; 115-124.

Sharpe P (1992). Comparative effects of bilateral hand splints and an elbow orthosis on stereotypic hand movements and toy play in two children with Rett syndrome. *Amer. J. Occ. Ther.* 46; 134-140.

Shea S, Turgay A, Carroll A, Schulz M, Orlik H, Smith I, Dunbar F (2004). Risperidone in the treatment of disruptive behavioural symptoms in children with autistic and other pervasive developmental disorders. *Paediatrics* 114; e634-e641.

Siminoff E, Stores G (1987). Controlled trial of trimeprazine tartrate for night-waking. *Archives of Disease in Childhood* 62; 253-257.

Simpson D, Gracies J, Graham H, et al., (2008). Assessment: Botulinum neurotoxin for the treatment of spasticity (an evidence-based review): report of the therapeutics and technology assessment subcommittee of the American Academy of Neurology. *Neurology* 70; 1691-1698.

Stenborn Y, Tonnby B, Hagberg B (1998). Lamotrigine in Rett syndrome: treatment experience from a pilot study. *Eur. Child Adolesc. Psych.*. 7(1):49-52.

Tarquino D, Motil K, Hou W, Lee H, Glaze D, Skinner S, Neul J, Annese F, McNair L, Barrish J, Geerts S, Lane J, Percy A (2012). Growth failure and outcome in Rett syndrome. *Neurol* 79(16); 1653-1661.

Temudo T, Rios M, Prior C, Carilho I, Santos M, Maciel P, Sequeiro J, Fonseca M, Monteiro J, Cabral P, Vieira J, Ormazabal A, Artuch R (2009). Evaluation of CSF neurotransmitters and folate in 25 patients with Rett disorder and effects of treatment. *Brain Dev.* 31; 46–51

Thommessen M, Kase B, Heiberg A (2008). Growth and nutrition in 10 girls with Rett syndrome.

Tropea D, Giacometti E, Wilson N, Beard C, McCurry C, Fu D, Flannery R, Jaenisch R, Sur M (2009). Partial reversal of Rett syndrome-like symptoms in MeCP2 mutant mice. *PNAS* 106(6); 2029-2034.

Toward M, Abdala A, Knopp S, Paton F, Bissonnette J (2013). Increasing brain serotonin corrects CO_2 chemosensitivity in methyl-CpG-binding protein MECP2)- deficient mice. *Exper Physiol.* 98(3); 842-849.

Van Esch H, Bauters M, Ignatius J, Jansen M, Reynaud M, Hollanders K, Lugtenberg D, Bienvenu T, Jensen L, Gecz J, Moraine C, Marynen P, Fryns JP, Froyen G (2005). Duplication of the MECP2 Region Is a Frequent Cause of Severe Mental Retardation and Progressive Neurological Symptoms in Males. *Am. J. Hum. Genet.* 77; 442-453.

Viemari J, Roux J, Tryba A, Saywell V, Burnet H, Peña F, Zanella S, Bévengut M, Barthelemy-Requin M, Herzing L, Moncla A, Mancini J, Ramirez JM, Villard L, Hilaire G (2005). Mecp2 deficiency disrupts norepinephrine and respiratory systems in mice. *J. Neurosci.* 25(50); 11521-11530.

Voituron N, Hilaire G (2011). The benzodiazepine Midazolam mitigates the breathing defects in Mecp2-deficient mice. *Respir. Physiol. Neurobiol.* 177; 56-60.

Wang H. Chan S, Ogier M, Hellard D, Wang Q, Smith C, Katz D (2006). Dysregulation of brain-derived neurotrophic factor expression and neurosecretory function in Mecp2-null mice. *J. Neurosci.* 26; 10911-10915.

Wang-Weigand S, McCue M, Ogrinc F, Mini L (2009). Effects of ramelton 8mg on objective sleep latency in adults with chronic insomnia on nights 1 and 2; a pooled analysis. *Curr. Med. Res. Opin.* 25; 1209-1213.

Weaving L, Ellaway C, Gecz J, Christodoulou J (2005). Rett syndrome: clinical review and molecular update. *J. Med. Genet.* 42: 1-7.

Weese-Mayer D, Lieske S, Boothby C, Kenny A, Bennett H, Silvestri J, Ramirez J (2006). Autonomic nervous system dysregulation : Breathing and heart rate perturbation during wakefulness in young girls with Rett syndrome. *Paediatr. Res.* 60; 443-449.

Welch E, Barton E, Zhuo J, Tomizawa Y, Friesen W, Trifillis P, Paushkin S, Patel M, Trotta C, Hwang S et al., (2007). PTC124 targets genetic disorders caused by nonsense mutations. *Nature* 447; 87-91.

Weng S, McLeod F, Bailey M, Cobb S (2011). Synaptic plasticity deficits in an experimental model of Rett syndrome: long-term potentiation saturation and its pharmacological reversal. *Neurosci.* 180; 314-321.

Wenk G, Mobley S (1996). Choline acetyltransferase activity and vesamicol binding in Rett syndrome and in rats with nucleus basalis lesions. *Neurosci* 73; 79-84.

Wigram T, Lawrence M (2005). Music therapy as a toll for assessing hand use and communicativeness in children with Rett syndrome. *Brian Dev.* 27; S95-S96.

Wilfong AA, Schultz RJ (2006). Vagus nerve stimulation for treatment of epilepsy in Rett syndrome. *Dev. Med. Child Neurol.* 48(8): 683-6.

Wilken B, Lally P, Bischoff A et al., (1997). Treatment of apneustic respiratory disturbance with a serotonin receptor agonist. *J. Paediatr* 130; 47-54.

Williams K, Brignell A, Randall M, Silove N, Hazell P (2013). Selective serotonin reuptake inhibitors (SSRIs) for autism spectrum disorders (ASD). *Cochrane Database Syst Rev*. CD004677.

Woo R (2001). Spasticity: Orthopaedic perspectives. *J. Child Neurol.* 16; 47-53.

Wood L, Gray N, Zhou Z, Greenberg M, Shepherd G (2009). Synaptic circuit abnormalities of motor-frontal 2/3 pyramidal neurons in an RNA interference model of methyl-CpG-binding protein 2 deficiency. *J. Neurosci.* 29; 12440-12448.

Wood L, Shepherd G (2010). Synaptic circuit abnormalities of motor-frontal layer 2/3 pyramidal neurons in a mutant mouse model of Rett syndrome. *Neurobiol. Dis.*. 38; 281-287.

Young D, Hong E, Castle J, Crespo-Barreto J, Bowman A, Rose M, Kang D, Richman R, Johnson J, Berget S, Zoghbi H (2005). Regulation of RNA splicing by the methylation-dependent transcriptional repressor methyl-CpG-binding protein 2. *PNAS USA* 102; 17551-17558.

Yvan V, Rudolph C, Lorenzo C, Hassall E, Liptak G, Mazur L, Sondheimer J, Staiano A, Thomson M, Veereman-Wauters G, Wenzyl T (2009). Pediatric Gastroesophageal Reflux Clinical Practice Guidelines: Joint Recommendations of the North American Society for Pediatric Gastroenterology, Hepatology, and Nutrition (NASPGHAN) and the European Society for Pediatric Gastroenterology, Hepatology, and Nutrition (ESPGHAN). *J. Pediatr Gastroenterol. Nutr.*, 49(4) 498-547.

Zammit G, Erman M, Wang-Weigand S, Sainati S, Zhang J, Roth T (2007). Evaluation of the efficacy and safety of ramelton in subjects with chronic insomnia. *J. Clin. Sleep Med.* 3; 495-504.

Zanella S, Mebarek S, Lajard AM, Picard N, Dutchsman M, Hilaire G (2008). Oral treatment with desipramine improves breathing and life span in Rett syndrome mouse model. *Resp. Physiol. Neurobiol.* 160; 116-121.

Zapella M (1990). A double blind trial of bromocriptine in the Rett syndrome. *Brain Dev*12(1):148-50.

Zhang L, He J, Jugloff D, Eubanks J (2008). The Mecp2 null mouse hippocampus displays altered basal inhibitory rhythms and is prone to hyperexcitability. *Hippocampus* 18; 294-309.

Zheng W, Quirion R (2004). Comparative signalling pathways of insulin-like growth factor and brain-derived neurotrophic factor in hippocampal neurons and the role of the PI3 kinase pathway in cell survival. *J. Neurochem.* 89; 844-852.

Zhou Z, Hong E, Cohen S, Zhao W, Ho H, Schmidt L, Chen W, Lin Y, Savner E, Griffith E, Hu L, Steen J, Weitz C, Greenberg M (2006). Brain-specific phosphorylation of MeCP2 regulates activity-dependent BDNF transcription, dendritic growth and spine maturation. *Neuron* 52; 255-269.

In: Rett Syndrome and Other Communication ... ISBN: 978-1-63463-920-0
Editor: Daniel L. Kolby

Chapter 2

Assistive Technology to Promote Communication, Leisure and Occupation Skills for Children with Rett Syndrome and Severe to Profound Developmental Disabilities: A Literature Overview

***Fabrizio Stasolla*[1,*] *and Viviana Perilli*[2]**
[1]Lega del Filo d'Oro Research Center, Molfetta, Italy
[2]Lega del Filo d'Oro Research Center, Lesmo, italy

Abstract

This chapter provides a literature overview concerning empirical studies aimed at promoting adaptive behaviors (e.g. communicative skills, locomotion) and reducing stereotypic behaviors (e.g. body rocking, hand clipping) in children with Rett syndrome and severe to profound developmental disabilities through rehabilitative programs based on

* Corresponding Author: Fabrizio Stasolla (e-mail: f.stasolla@psico.uniba.it, f.stasolla@libero.it).

cognitive-behavioral interventions and/or assistive technology, published in the last period (i.e. 2000-2014). A combined computerized and manual search was conducted to identify the empirical evidences that were retained for the overview. That is, 20 studies were selected for this purpose. Outcomes were largely positive and encouraging, although some failure occurred. A second goal of the chapter was to point out strengths and weakness of the aforementioned studies. Finally, a third objective was to emphasize critical issues and future questions to be addressed for the future research and practice in this topic area. Clinical, educational and psychological implications of the findings are also discussed.

Keywords: Rett syndrome, assistive technology, quality of life, indices happiness, developmental disabilities, adaptive behaviors

1. Introduction

Rett syndrome (RS) is a progressive neurodevelopmental disorder, X linked, due to genetic mutations in the methyl-cytosine phosphsate-guanine binding protein 2 (MECP2) gene, located on Xq28 chromosome, affecting primarily females, first described by Andreas Rett (Rett, 1966). It includes a gradual loss of cognitive, communicative, and motor functions, beginning between 6 and 18 month, following an apparent normal birth and an initial regular development (Stasolla & Caffò, 2013). RS is commonly characterized by four main stages such as: (a) stagnation, (b) regression, (c) stationary, and (d) motor deterioration (Didden et al., 2010; Stasolla, De Pace, et al., 2014). During stagnation, starting between 5 and 6 months, a general arrest of child's development and adaptive skills are observed.. The second stage (i.e. regression) has an onset between 1 and 4 years old (Sigafoos et al., 2009) and presents a decline of communicative functions (i.e. speech and language), although eye contact (i.e. gazing) is relatively preserved. The Stationary (third) stage emphasizes hand stereotyped behaviors such as mouthing, washing and clapping, added to breath abnormalities (i.e. hyperventilation) and nocturne behavioral disturbances (i.e. laughing and crying). Furthermore, apraxia, ataxia, motor scoliosis and seizures are included, between 2 and 10 years old (Young et al., 2011). The final fourth stage (i.e. motor deterioration) is described with physical impairments, reduced mobility, and decreased stereotypic movements, after 10 years old (Marschik, 2013). Revised criteria by Neul e al. (2010) include severe to profound intellectual and developmental disabilities, withdrawal, failing of ambulation responses. Children with RS are usually very isolated and passive, displaying minimal capacities to interact positively with the surrounding world. Moreover, they exhibit very limited adaptive behaviors, reduced sensory inputs, passivity and they are often described as extremely sedentary, with negative consequences on their quality of life (Felce & Perry, 1995; Ivancic & Bailey, 1996). The complexity of their clinical conditions may pose serious problems to parents, staff and caregivers, while dealing with improving constructive engagement and positive mood for those children, within home, school, and/or rehabilitative settings (Lancioni, Singh, O'Reilly, Oliva, & Basili, 2005). One way to ensure children with RS by promoting self-determination, constructive engagement and consequently prevent their withdrawal and isolation, is the use of assistive technology (Lancioni, Sigafoos, O'Reilly, & Singh, 2012; Lancioni & Singh, 2014).

Beside a large body of literature concerning rehabilitative interventions aimed at enhancing communicative functions by children with RS (Fabio, Antonietti, Castelli, & Marchetti, 2009; Sigafoos et al., 2009, 2011; Stasolla, De Pace, et al., 2014), there is a wide empirical evidence (Fabio et al., 2013; Lancioni et al., 2014; Lotan & Gootman, 2012) describing programs designed at improving adaptive social functions such as occupation, reduction of stereotypic behaviors, increasing locomotion. Furthermore, a relevant topic in this research area is to monitor and assess the effects of the aforementioned interventions on the indices of happiness of the participants involved, as a sign of positive mood and quality of life (Lancioni et al., 2005).

The first goal of this chapter is to provide a general picture of the empirical studies published between 2000 and 2014, concerning the assistive technologies developed at improving self-determination, constructive engagement, and occupation skills by children with RS. Next to the attention given to communicative functions, studies included in this overview will consider the overall adaptive functions regarding children with RS such as independent access to preferred stimuli, choice opportunities, locomotion fluency, in order to underline the most recent strategies and rehabilitative interventions applied to children with RS and using AT based on learning principles (i.e. association between a behavioral response and an environmental consequence). Moreover, the chapter will emphasize empirical evidences aimed at reducing stereotypic behaviors exhibited by children with RS as well as studies dealing with the effects on positive mood. The second purpose of the chapter is to underline strengths and weaknesses of the different studies included in the overview.

Finally, the third objective is to point out critical issues and questions to be addressed in the future and to discuss their clinical, psychological and rehabilitative implications for research and practice.

2. Method

A computerized search was performed in electronic databases such as SCOPUS, PUBMED, ERIC, and PSYCHINFO, by inserting Rett syndrome, developmental disabilities, quality of life, indices of happiness, cognitive-behavioural interventions, assistive technology, adaptive behaviours, stereotypic behaviours, communication impairments, social skills, self-determination, constructive engagement and their combination as keywords. A manual search was also completed in order to integrate such identification. Including criteria concerned: (a) at least one child or adolescent (i.e. age range 0-19 years) with RS involved, (b) at least one cognitive-behavioural intervention approach and/or an assistive technology-based program, and (c) at least an outcome measure of quality of life. Excluding criteria considered: (a) studies published before 2000, (b) theoretical and/or assessment/descriptive studies (i.e. without any empirical evidence and/or without introducing any rehabilitative program/technique), (c) studies aimed at investigating the neuro-physiological, bio-molecular, and/or genetic substrate, with any behavioural issue, and (d) articles published differently from English language. Following the aforementioned criteria, 20 studies were retained, including 172 participants.

For practical reasons, studies were grouped in three main categories (i.e. enhancing communicative functions, reducing stereotypic behaviours, fostering locomotion), depending on their rehabilitative goals. Moreover, irrespective of the number of studies included in each of the aforementioned categories, three empirical evidences will be synthetically described within each group, pointing out the number of participants involved, their behavioural characteristics with their ages, the rehabilitative purposes, the procedures adopted and the results carried out, were available. For a complete overview of the selected studies readers may refer to table 1.

3. Summaries of the Studies Included in the Overview

3.1. Improving Communications Skills of Children with RS

In light of the above mentioned characteristics of children with RS, one of the critical rehabilitative goal is the improvement of communicative functions concerning those individuals.

Table 1. Studies grouped according to their rehabilitative goals

Studies	Participants	Age Ranges	Responses	Outcomes
Communicative Skills				
Koppenhaver et al., 2002	6	3-6	Read a story	Six positive
Ryan et al., 2004	3	9.1-16.2	Toy play	Three positive
Baptista et al., 2006	7	4.1-9.6	Eye gazing	Three negative
Hetzroni & Rubin, 2006	8	6-11	Eye gazing	Eight positive
Djukic et al., 2012	44	4-16	Visual fixation	Nine negative
Byiers et al., 2014	1	15	Functional Training	One positive
Stasolla et al., 2014	3	8.4-10.5	Select and choose items	Three positive
Stereotypic Behaviors				
Shetty et al., 2000	1	12	Hand movements	One positive
Wales et al., 2004	8	5-18	Hand movements	Six positive
Temudo et al., 2007	1	2	Hand/limb movements	One positive
Nissenkorn & Ben-Zeev, 2013	5	6-15	Hand tapping	Five positive
Quest et al., 2013	4	12-18	Hand stereotypy	Four positive
Stasolla & Caffò, 2013	2	12-17	Body rocking	Two positive
Stasolla et al., 2015	3	9.8-12.4	Mouthing/washing	Three positive
Ambulation/Locomotion				
Lotan et al., 2004	4	8.5-11	Physical exercise	Four positive
Shapiro et al., 2010	49	1.9-17	Ambulation	Forty five positive
Castelli et al., 2013	9	5-19	Step responses	Nine positive
Stasolla & Caffò, 2013	2	12-17	Locomotion fluency	Two positive

Table 1. (Continued)

Studies	Participants	Age Ranges	Responses	Outcomes
Isaias et al., 2014	11	6-12	Gait initiation	Eleven positive
Schaefer & Johnson (in press)	1	5	Ambulation	One positive

Thus, by enhancing communicative skills, one may prevent deprivation, withdrawal and foster the participation of children with RS within daily contexts, facilitating their social interactions with peers, teachers, parents and caregivers. Furthermore, their independence will be performed, with positive consequences and beneficial effects on their social desirability, image and status (Stasolla et al., 2015). That is, children with RS will be able to communicate their needs autonomously, with a reduction of caregivers' burden (Mc grew & Keyes, 2014). Studies on this topic research area are critically focused on (a) increasing participants' responsiveness to vocalizations, body movements and/or eye gazing concerning existing persons in the surrounding environment, (b) teaching the use of new communicative strategies such as graphics symbols, pictograms, vocal output communication aids (VOCAs) and/or speech generating devices (SGDs), (c) augmenting individual participation in interactions with social partners, and (d) improving initiatives and/or requests to one or more communicative partners (Sigafoos et al., 2009, 2011). Overall, 7 studies involving 72 participants are included in this section (see table 1 for a complete overview).

For example, Stasolla, De Pace, et al. (2014) carried out a study aimed at the systematic comparison between PECS and VOCA strategies for enhancing communication skills of three girls with RS. The participants, aged of 9.2, 8.4, and 10.5 (mean age of 9.36), and received a diagnosis of RS at 20, 16 and 18 months old respectively. They were reported with severe communication impairments (i.e. lack of speech, although they were capable of some vocalizations), seizures, hyperventilation, withdrawal, stereotypic behaviours (i.e. body rocking, tipping and washing hand-related movements), profound developmental disabilities, failing in locomotion. The study was conducted according to an alternating treatments design, where the two aforementioned communicative strategies (i.e. PECS and VOCA) were first learned singly, then combined together. Results pointed out that all children involved increased their communicative skills and reduced their stereotyped behaviours with beneficial effects on their positive mood (i.e. indices of happiness) with both strategies during intervention phases compared to baselines. Moreover, two of them always chose VOCA intervention within the preference checks assessment phase, while the third girl equally selected both treatments.

Byiers, Dimian and Symons (2014) worked on an adolescent with RS who was 15 years old at the beginning of the study. The participant was exposed to a functional communication training combined with a functional assessment in order to teach new communicative behaviour. By using single-case experimental design, functional reinforcements were selected, aimed at learning of a VOCA's activation useful to obtain a preferred environmental event, through the caregiver's mediation. Results showed an increasing of the participant's performance during the training sessions, which pointed out that individuals with RS may acquire new communicative responses, with positive implications for future research and practice.

Koppenhaver et al. (2001) used a storybook-based communication intervention for six girls with RS for improving their communication abilities while interacting with their mothers. The participants, aged from 3 to 7 years old, presented severe communication impairments and lack of intelligible speech. They all communicated with nonconventional modes such as gestures and vocalizations. Furthermore, their communicative capacities were based on gaze orientation concerning a desired object. Moreover, they were all reported within the severe to profound range of intellectual disabilities from school personnel. The objective of the study was to provide a natural language learning context, in which early communication was positive reinforced and supported. Effects of resting hand splints, light technology augmentative communication such as VOCA/symbols and basic parent trainings and symbolic communication and labelling behaviours for the six girls were observed within home contexts, while reading familiar and unfamiliar stories with their mothers. Results showed that all girls became more active and sympathetic in the interactions during storybook reading. They all employed a wide range of communication modes, increasing their labelling capacities. Moreover, three of them improved their performance during familiar stories reading compared to unfamiliar ones.

3.2. Reducing Stereotypic Behaviours in Children with RS

A second peculiarity of children with RS is undoubtedly represented by stereotypic behaviours such as body rocking, hand clapping, hand tipping and hand washing as consequence of the progressive loss of their functionality.

Moreover, the self-stimulation (i.e. stereotyped behaviours) is one (aberrant) way to prevent deprivation by those individuals. Within this topic area, rehabilitative programs are aimed at pursuing the dual goal of enhancing (i.e. positive reinforcing) an adaptive behaviour and reducing a challenge behaviour (e.g. hand mouthing). Behavioural interventions may include different techniques and/or strategies such as response blocking, mechanical restraints, differential reinforcement of alternative behaviours (i.e. DRA), modelling, shaping, hypercorrection, non-contingent reinforcement, microswitch-cluster (Lancioni, Singh, O'Reilly, & Sigafoos, 2009). Seven studies are retained in this section, involving 24 participants (see table 1).

For example, Quest, Byiers, Payen and Symons (2014) exposed five girls with RS (mean age 17.8) to direct behavioural observation to measure the amount of hand stereotypic behaviours of negative affect during periods of high and low stress conditions. Results showed that negative affect occurred more likely during high stress conditions, while hand stereotypic behaviours did not significantly differ across conditions. Therefore, hand stereotypic behaviour did not seem to be a predictor of stress responses in girls with RS. Alternatively, stress conditions were not sufficiently stronger as to evoke the exhibition of hand stereotypic behaviours.

Stasolla et al. (2015) exposed three girls with RS ranging from 9 to 12 years old (mean age 10.83) to an assistive technology-based program aimed at promoting occupation and choice strategies on one hand and at increasing indices o happiness and reducing stereotypic behaviours on the other. The study was carried out according to a multiple probe design across behaviours, where the three adaptive behaviours were first learned singly and subsequently combined together. Results emphasized an improvement of the performance and a decreasing of stereotyped behaviours for all participants involved during intervention phases compared to baselines.

Stasolla and Caffò (2013) worked on two girls with RS (aged of 12 and 17 years respectively) applying a microswitch-based program aimed at promoting object manipulation and reducing stereotypic behaviours. Moreover, the effects of the rehabilitative program on indices of happiness of the participants were monitored. Since two adaptive behaviours were learned, the study was carried out according to a multiple probe design across behaviours for both participants involved. The two girls increased their adaptive responses and decreased their stereotypic behaviours during intervention phases compared to baselines.

3.3. Promoting Ambulation Responses in Children with RS

Children with RS and severe to profound developmental disabilities may exhibit problems of balance with negative consequences on their gait process, ambulation responses and locomotion fluency (Lancioni et al., 2010). The first common approach used to deal with such difficulty rely on neuro-developmental strategy widely based on Bobath 's model, which point out the relevance of inhibiting abnormal body movements and promoting postural corrections, involving the therapist-direct practice of motor responses or tasks, while the child is lying, sitting or standing (Bobath & Bobath, 1984). Conversely, new intervention approaches within this topic area underline the child-centered (i.e. active role) of task-specific practice as a crucial issue for enhancing the targeted motor behaviours (Lancioni, et al., 2010). According to this view, it is critical for fostering and performing the ambulation responses, enabling the child to positively practice such responses. A first traditional approach consists of the use of treadmills combined with partial body weight balancing (i.e. support). A second nonconventional strategy may be represented by the use of microswitches combined with walkers and contingent positive stimulation (Lancioni et al., 2013). That is, based on learning principles (i.e. association between a behavioural step response and preferred high desirable contingent environmental events) the child would learn to improve his/her gait process (Lancioni et al., 2004). Six studies were retained in this section including 76 participants.

For example, Lotan, Isakov, & Merrick (2004) conducted a study on 4 girls with RS (ranging age 8.5-11 years old) to investigate the feasibility of a physical exercise program to promote fitness and health, through the use of treadmills. Specifically, the training with the treadmill was carried out on an educational facility, on a 1400 model treadmill (i.e. Trimline, capable of low speed such as <0.5 km/h), with very long side rails. The side rails' adaptation facilitated the fitness of children' height and at the same time Velcro straps were inserted in order to assist participants in placing their hands. Pulses were measured during the exercise though the use of a polar pulse belt. Functional monitoring was carried out with the mediation of a 31-items sale adopted for the study concerning the knee walk, the knee stand, the participants' ability to get up (i.e. standing position), the duration of different walking paths, and the capacity to go up and down stairs. Results showed that the physical fitness of all children involved in the study was greatly (i.e. statistically significant) grown at the end of the training program. Moreover, all children improved their motor abilities, with positive consequences on their general health and fitness conditions.

Isaias et al. (2014) investigated the anticipatory of postural adjustments linked to gait initiation by 11 girls with RS (ranging age from 6 to 12 years old) compared to 10 health girls. The outcomes measures concerned the recording of muscles activities (i.e. tibialis anterior and soleus), ground reaction forces and body kinematic. Experimental group (i.e. the 11 girls with RS) emphasized a temporal organization impairment, added to a diminished impulse to move forward underlined by a deficit in several parameters concerning the starting gait process such as length and rapidity of the first step, magnitude and orientation of centre of centre-pressure of mass vector contingently with the swing-toe off. Data allowed to underline abnormalities associated with the muscular pattern activation which was featured by a disruption on the functioning of antagonistic pairs of postural muscles in individuals with RS.

Stasolla and Caffò (2013) exposed two adolescents (i.e. aged of 12 and 17 years old respectively) to a microswitch-based program aimed at promoting locomotion fluency (i.e. following a basic criterion of performing 4 forward steps within 3 seconds). Experimental conditions were planned according to a multiple probe design across behaviours (since the locomotion fluency was combined with an independent access to preferred stimuli through object manipulation, see above). Both girls improved their performance (i.e. locomotion fluency) during intervention phases compared to baselines. Furthermore, the rehabilitative program showed beneficial effects on positive mood (i.e. indices of happiness) for both adolescents involved.

4. Discussion

Overall, data collected in the studies selected for this overview showed that assistive technology-based programs and cognitive-behavioural interventions were successful and useful for children with RS, by enhancing their adaptive responses, improving their communicative skills, fostering their gait process and ambulation responses, reducing their stereotypic behaviours, and increasing their positive mood and constructive engagement. These findings, largely supported by research literature reviews concerning this topic area (Go, 2007; Moss & Howlin, 2009; Muhle, Trentacoste, & Rapin, 2004; Shea, 2004) underline the feasibility, the suitability and the affordability of such strategies for individuals with RS and severe to profound developmental disabilities, suggesting the following considerations.

First, cognitive-behavioural interventions and assistive technology-based programs may be accounted as great and crucial educational and rehabilitative resources in order to promote self-determination, central and active role, positive participation and direct involvement of children with RS. That is, by enabling children with RS to interact positively with the surrounding world, one may envisage their commitment and high motivation in selecting and choosing their access independently (i.e. without caregiver's mediation) to preferred events. Thus, one may argue that within this approach children with RS reduce their passivity, prevent withdrawal and isolation with positive consequences no their social image, desirability and status, by improving constructive engagement of those individuals. Moreover, the aforementioned strategies may represent a basic approach with clinical implications for research and practice (Lancioni, Sigafoos, O'Reilly, & Singh, 2012; Lancioni & Singh, 2014; Stasolla et al., 2015; Stasolla & Caffò, 2013; Stasolla, De Pace, et al., 2014).

Second, by enhancing their communicative skills, improving their locomotion behaviour and gait process, and reducing their stereotyped behaviours, children with RS are more easily integrated in social contexts such as home, medical, rehabilitative and school settings, with a significant reduction of caregivers' burden (Mulroy, Robertson, Aiberti, Leonard, & Bower, 2008). Precisely, children with RS will be enabled to communicate their needs, to improve their opportunities of request and choice desired items and to receive those items automatically through the technological system or with the mediation of the caregiver. Furthermore, by increasing their constructive engagement, occupation and leisure skills in such activities, they would reduce their necessity of self-stimulation, with positive consequences on their quality of life (Lancioni, Singh, O'Reilly, Oliva, & Basili, 2005; Matson, Fodstad, & Boisjoli, 2008; Matson & LoVullo, 2009; Matson & Sipes, 2010). Next to their integration, children with RS and severe to profound developmental disabilities would acquire new adaptive responses, ensuring them with positive (external and/or environmental) reinforcements (Lancioni et al., 2014; Marschik, Einspieler, & Sigafoos, 2012; Marschik et al., 2014).

Third, a customer-tailored intervention program such as those used in the studies reviewed is significantly relevant for any child with RS and pervasive developmental disabilities. Therefore, by designing a treatment with solution adopted strictly for one person and varying their applicability depending on their usage for other individuals provide their suitability and affordability for different children with RS and/or other developmental disabilities. Moreover, often their costs are limited (i.e. cheap or not expensive) and they could consequently be adopted for a large numbers of users, constituting and representing, once more, an essential way to operate in several contexts and/or environmental conditions (Lancioni, Comes, et al., 2005; Stasolla, Perilli, & Damiani, 2014; Stasolla, Damiani, & Caffò, 2014). Furthermore, their constant and continuous updating according the complexity of the participants upon their characteristics and/or clinical conditions due to their pathology is undoubtedly mandatory (Brown, Schalock, & Brown, 2009; Dillon & Carr, 2007; Reichle, 2011).

Fourth, almost all participants involved in the different studies seemed to enjoy the sessions, with an increasing of their indices of happiness during the intervention phases compared to baselines. Moreover, participants consolidated their enjoyment during maintenance, follow-up and post intervention check phases, where available. Thus, by varying systematically positive events as reinforcements for adaptive responses learned by participants, one may encourage constructive engagement, positive participation and high motivation preventing saturation, with positive consequences on their quality of life (Lancioni, Singh, O'Reilly, Oliva, & Basili, 2005). Since participants maintain their performance over the time, one may argue that the proposed intervention strategies adopted are effective and useful in improving positive mood of participants involved (De Pace & Stasolla, 2014; Federici & Scherer, 2012).

Fifth, stereotypic behaviours were significantly reduced during interventions phases. That is, by being constructive engaged, high motivated and positively reinforced by contingent stimulation delivered by the system to adaptive responses, participants did not require to stimulate by them-selves, spending less time exhibiting stereotyped responses. Furthermore, their social desirability and general environmental acceptance (i.e. social image and status) were substantially increased, once more with beneficial effects on their quality of life (De Pace & Stasolla, 2015; Matson, 2012; Matson & Sturmey, 2011; Stasolla et al., 2015).

Sixth, interventions validity (i.e. clinical and practical) was robustly corroborated by maintenance/generalization phases and preference checks and/or social validation assessment, where available. That is, either participants directly involved (i.e. through preference checks) and external raters (i.e. with social validation) confirmed the effectiveness of the rehabilitative programs designed within the studies reviewed. Thus, both internal (i.e. participants involved) and external (i.e. social validation raters) provided a formal endorsement concerning the aforementioned strategies (Caffò, et al., 2014; Lancioni et al., 2006; Stasolla, Perilli, & Damiani, 2014).

Seventh, positive outcomes and success of an assistive technology-based program would widely depend on four main features: (a) behavioural response(s) selected and requested by the participant, (b) positive stimulation retained as reinforcement, (c) technological solutions adopted, and (d) cover (i.e. be extended) over the day (Lancioni, Singh, O'Reilly, & Oliva, 2005). With regard to the behavioural response selected, one should consider the one easily produced by the participant within his/her repertoire (i.e. exhibited without effort), exhibited with external prompt (i.e. physical, verbal or both simultaneously), objectively measurable, and affordably detected by the technological solution (e.g. microswitch). With regard to the positive stimulation, it should be high motivating and systematically varied within the same designed study. In fact, by selecting high motivating (i.e. pleasant) stimuli to be used as reinforcements, one may significantly reduce the response cost for the participant (i.e. the fatigue required to produce and exhibit the behavioural response) and by varying systematically the positive reinforcements, saturation is relevantly prevented. Finally, by extending the amount of the time across the day and by repeating it along the week, the rehabilitative intervention may represent a crucial educational and psychological approach in order to envisage for children with RS and developmental disabilities high motivating contexts (Lancioni et al., 2014; Stasolla et al., 2015).

Eighth, it is high desirable to design different rehabilitative programs having various educational goals within the same studies and the same experimental conditions (Kennedy, 2005). For example, one may provide children with RS with a microswitch and VOCA (i.e. speech generating device, SGD) ensuring the children involved with independent access to preferred stimulation (i.e. microswitch) and/or asking for social contact with a caregiver (i.e. VOCA) (Lancioni et al., 2009). Otherwise, one may consider to enable children with RS with the to look for pleasant stimulation on one hand, and promoting ambulation responses or fostering locomotion fluency on the other (Stasolla & Caffò, 2013). Else, one may encounter for one or more microswitch cluster-based program aimed at enhancing an adaptive response and diminishing a challenge behaviour (Stasolla et al., 2014). Finally, one may use computer assisted-based program in order to promote choice behaviours (Stasolla, Caffò, Picucci, & Bosco, 2013).

Conclusion

In light of above, one may argue that assistive technology-based programs may be considered as a basic crucial resource to ensure children with RS with self-determination, constructive engagement, positive participation, preventing isolation, withdrawal and passivity, with positive consequences on their quality of life. The solutions adopted within the studies selected for this overview seemed to be effective and useful in this way. Depending on the rehabilitative goals and objectives, one may design some intervention strategy instead of other, as pointed out and stated above. Although most of the reviewed studies emphasized positive outcomes, some failure occurred and it is in order to avoid those failures that one should envisage some corrections, dealing with the following four perspectives for the future research.

First, the continuous updating and extension of such technologies to new participants with RS responding to their complexity and clinical conditions is undoubtedly necessary. The medical evolution (i.e. history) of the participants involved should be always be examined. Moreover, finding new (and eventually) non-typical behavioural responses to be selected for the use of assistive technologies adopted should represent a primary purpose for the future research (Lancioni, Singh, O'Reilly, & Sigafoos, 2009; Lancioni et al., 2007; Stasolla et al., 2014). Furthermore, a rigorous systematic variation of the stimulation in order to provide participants with a wide range of reinforcements and opportunities of choice is equally critical and essential (Lancioni & Singh, 2014). For example, one may consider the use of an i-pad with a touch screen and different options automatically scanned with a double (i.e. visual and verbal) presentation to ensure children with RS to communicate their needs (Sigafoos et al., 2013). Else, one may envisage a microswitch-based program compared to a treadmill-based intervention in order to systematically alternate two different strategies within the same experimental design, as reported above (Barlow, Nock, & Hersen, 2009).

Second, the definition, the description and the assessment of practical guidelines concerning the rehabilitative programs and interventions should be highly encouraged, specifically to prevent the aforementioned failures. That is, one should precise contextual conditions in order to promote adaptive responses, reduce stereotypic behaviours, improve positive participation, enhance commitment and motivation by participants involved, reducing parents and/or caregivers' burden. Moreover, one may envisage the integration of such programs with more traditional/conventional ones such as stimulation sessions, speech sessions and/or physiotherapy, aimed at the inclusion of children with RS in daily contexts (e.g. home, school, medical or rehabilitative settings) (Lancioni, Sigafoos, O'Reilly, & Singh, 2012).

Third, one should design research projects and/or interventions useful to concretely activate the aforementioned guidelines, without excessive requests and efforts by staff and caregivers. Thus, usually educational and medical centres (e.g. school context) may not have adequate resources for complete monitoring of those strategies and may rely on more traditional restraints. For this goal, one may envisage cheap (i.e. not expensive) technological solutions and sensorial inputs not demanding high cost by personnel (Federici & Scherer, 2012).

Fourth, future research should extend the clinical validity of such interventions, by using more systematically social validation assessment involving parents, professionals, support teachers, and students as raters, in order to further endorse the rehabilitative programs. Furthermore, in order to assess the history of participants involved, one may argue that preference checks, maintenance, generalization and follow-up phases should be always strictly recommended, even if contextual condition do not allow their satisfactory realization (e.g. school, home and medical settings do not provide their implementation) (Kazdin, 2001). Thus, the aforementioned endorsement is crucial for the effectiveness, the affordability, the suitability and the plausibility of an assistive technology-based intervention for children with severe to profound developmental disabilities, irrespective of their pathology (e.g. Rett syndrome) (Barlow, Andrasik, & Hersen, 2006).

References

Baptista, P. M., Mercadante, M. T., Macedo, E. C., & Schwartzman, J. S. (2006). Cognitive performance in Rett syndrome girls: A pilot study using eyetracking technology. *Journal of Intellectual Disability Research*, 50, 662-666.

Barlow, D. H., Andrasik, F., & Hersen, M. (2006). Single case experimental designs (3rd edition). Boston: *Allyn & Bacon*.

Barlow, D. H., Nock, M. K., & Hersen, M. (2009). Single-case experimental designs: *Strategies for studying behaviour change*. New York: Pearson.

Bobath, K., & Bobath, B. (1984). The neurodevelopmental treatment. In D. Scutton (Ed.), Management of the motor disorders of children with cerebral palsy. Clinics in developmental medicine no. 90 (pp. 6–18). London: *Spastic International Medical Publications*.

Brown, R.I., R.L. Schalock, R. L., & Brown, I. (2009). Q uality of Life: Its application to persons with intellectual disabilities and their families – Introduction and overview. *Journal of Policy & Practice in Intellectual Disabilities*, 6, 2-6.

Byiers, B. J., Dimian, A., & Symons, F. J. (2014). Functional communication training in Rett syndrome: A preliminary study. *American Journal of Intellectual and Developmental Disabilities*, 119, 340-350.

Caffò, A. O., Hoogeveen, F., Groenendaal, M., Perilli, V. A., Damen, M., Stasolla, F., et al. (2014). Comparing two different orientation strategies for promoting indoor traveling in people with alzheimer's disease. *Research in Developmental Disabilities*, 35, 572-580.

Castelli, I., Antonietti, A., Fabio, R. A., Lucchini, B., & Marchetti, A. (2013). Do Rett syndrome persons possess theory of mind? Some evidence from not-treated girls. *Life Span and Disability*, 16, 157-168.

Didden, R., Korzilius, H., Smeets, E., Green, V., Lang, R., Lancioni, G., et al. (2010). Communication in individuals with Rett syndrome: An assessment of forms and functions. *Journal of Developmental and Physical Disabilities*, 22, 105–118.

Dillon, C. M., & Carr, J. E. (2007). Assessing indices of happiness and unhappiness in individuals with developmental disabilities: A review. *Behavioral Interventions*, 22, 229-244.

Djukic, A., Valicenti McDermott, M., Mavrommatis, K., & Martins, C. L. (2012). Rett syndrome: Basic features of visual processing - A pilot study of eye-tracking. *Pediatric Neurology*, 47, 25-29.

Fabio, R. A., Antonietti, A., Castelli, I., & Marchetti, A. (2009). Attention and communication in Rett syndrome. *Research in Autism Spectrum Disorders,* 3, 329–335.

Fabio, R. A., Castelli, I., Marchetti, A., & Antonietti, A. (2013). Training communication abilities in rett syndrome through reading and writing. *Frontiers in Psychology*, 4(DEC).

Federici, S., & Scherer, M. (2012). Assistive technology assessment handbook. CRC Press.

Felce, D., & Perry, J. (1995). Quality of life: Its definition and measurement. *Research in Developmental Disabilities*,16, 51–74.

Go, T. (2007). Medical music therapy based on baby science (baby-science-based music therapy) and assistive technology for children. *Current Pediatric Reviews,* 3, 198-206.

Hetzroni, O. E., & Rubin, C. (2006). Identifying patterns of communicative behaviors in girls with rett syndrome. AAC: *Augmentative and Alternative Communication*, 22, 48-61.

Isaias, I. U., Dipaola, M., Michi, M., Marzegan, A., Volkmann, J., Roidi, M. L. R., et al. (2014). Gait initiation in children with rett syndrome. *PLoS* ONE, 9.

Ivancic, M. T., & Bayley, J. S. (1996). Current limits to reinforcement identification for some persons with profound multiple disabilities. *Research in Developmental Disabilities*, 17, 77–92.

Kazdin, A. E. (2001). Behavior modification in applied settings (6th edition). Belmont: Wadsworth.

Kennedy, C. H. (2005). Single case designs for educational research. Boston: *Allyn & Bacon.*

Koppenhaver, D. A., Erickson, K. A., Harris, B., McLellan, J., Skotko, B. G., & Newton, R. A. (2001). Storybook-based communication intervention for girls with Rett syndrome and their mothers. *Disability and Rehabilitation*, 23, 149-159.

Lancioni, G. E. Comes M. L., Stasolla F., Manfredi, F., O'Reilly M. F., Singh N. N., (2005). A Microswitch Cluster to Enhance Arm-Lifting Responses without Dystonic Head Tilting by a Child with Multiple Disabilities. *Perceptual and Motor Skills*, 100, 892-894.

Lancioni, G. E., & Singh, N. N. (2014). Assistive technologies for people with diverse abilities. New York: *Springer.*

Lancioni, G. E., O'Reilly, M. F., Singh, N. N., Groeneweg, J., Bosco, A., Tota, A., et al. (2006). A social validation assessment of microswitch-based programs for persons with multiple disabilities employing teacher trainees and parents as raters. *Journal of Developmental and Physical Disabilities*, 18, 383-391.

Lancioni, G. E., O'Reilly, M. F., Singh, N. N., Sigafoos, J., Didden, R., Oliva, D., et al. (2009). Persons with multiple disabilities accessing stimulation and requesting social contact via microswitch and VOCA devices: New research evaluation and social validation. *Research in Developmental Disabilities*, 30, 1084-1094.

Lancioni, G. E., Sigafoos, J., O'Reilly, M. F., & Singh, N. N. (2012). Assistive technology: Interventions for individuals with severe/profound and multiple disabilities. New York: *Springer.*

Lancioni, G. E., Singh, N. N., O'Reilly, M. F., & Oliva, D. (2005). Microswitch programs for persons with multiple disabilities: an overview of the responses adopted for microswitch activation. *Cognitive Processing* 6, 177-188.

Lancioni, G. E., Singh, N. N., O'Reilly, M. F., Oliva, D., & Basili, G. (2005). An overview of research on increasing indices of happiness of people with severe/profound intellectual and multiple disabilities. *Disability and Rehabilitation*, 27, 83–93.

Lancioni, G. E., Singh, N. N., O'Reilly, M. F., Sigafoos, J., Boccasini, A., La Martire, M. L. et al. (2014). Microswitch-aided programs for a woman with Rett Syndrome and a boy with extensive neuro-motor and intellectual disabilities. *Journal of Developmental and Physical Disabilities*, 26, 135-143.

Lancioni, G. E., Singh, N. N., O'Reilly, M. F., & Sigafoos, J. (2009). An overview of behavioral strategies for reducing hand-related stereotypies of persons with severe to profound intellectual and multiple disabilities: 1995-2007. *Research in Developmental Disabilities*, 30, 20-43.

Lancioni, G. E., Singh, N. N., O'Reilly, M. F., Oliva, D., Scalini, L., & Groeneweg, J. (2004). Improving assisted ambulation in a man with multiple disabilities through the use of a microswitch cluster. *Behavioural and Cognitive Psychotherapy*, 32, 245-249.

Lancioni, G. E., Singh, N. N., O'Reilly, M. F., Sigafoos, J., Chiapparino, C., Stasolla, F., et al. (2007). Enabling a young man with minimal motor behavior to manage independently his leisure television engagement. *Perceptual and Motor Skills*, 105, 47-54.

Lancioni, G. E., Singh, N. N., O'Reilly, M. F., Sigafoos, J., Oliva, D., Smaldone, A., et al. (2010). Promoting ambulation responses among children with multiple disabilities through walkers and microswitches with contingent stimuli. *Research in Developmental Disabilities*, 31, 811-816.

Lancioni, G. E., Singh, N. N., O'Reilly, M. F., Sigafoos, J., Oliva, D., Campodonico, F., & Buono, S. (2013). Walker devices and microswitch technology to enhance assisted indoor ambulation by persons with multiple disabilities: Three single-case studies. *Research in Developmental Disabilities*, 34, 2191-2199.

Lotan, M., & Gootman, A. (2012). Regaining walking ability in individuals with Rett syndrome: A case study. *International Journal on Disability and Human Development*, 11, 163–169.

Lotan, M., Isakov, E., & Merrick, J. (2004). Improving functional skills and physical fitness in children with rett syndrome. *Journal of Intellectual Disability Research*, 48, 730-735.

Marschik, P. B., Bartl-Pokorny, K. D., Tager-Flusberg, H., Kaufmann, W. E., Pokorny, F., Grossmann, T., et al. (2014). Three different profiles: Early socio-communicative capacities in typical Rett syndrome, the preserved speech variant and normal development. *Developmental Neurorehabilitation,* 17, 34-38.

Marschik, P. B., Einspieler, C., & Sigafoos, J. (2012). Contributing to the early detection of Rett syndrome: The potential role of auditory gestalt perception. *Research in Developmental Disabilities*, 33, 461-466.

Marschik, P. B., Kaufmann, W. E., Sigafoos, J., Wolin, T., Xhang, D., Bartl-Pokorny, K.D., et al. (2013). Changing the perspective on early development of Rett syndrome. *Research in Developmental Disabilities*, 34, 1236–1239.

Matson, J. L. (2012). Functional Assessment for Challenging Behaviors. New york: *Springer.*

Matson, J. L., & LoVullo, S. V. (2009). Trends and topics in autism spectrum disorders research. *Research in Autism Spectrum Disorders*, 3, 252-257.

Matson, J. L., & Sipes, M. (2010). Methods of early diagnosis and tracking for autism and pervasive developmental disorder not otherwise specified (PDDNOS). *Journal of Developmental and Physical Disabilities*, 22, 343-358.

Matson, J. L., & Sturmey, P. (2011). International Handbook of Autism and Pervasive Developmental Disorders. New York: *Springer.*

Matson, J. L., Fodstad, J. C., & Boisjoli, J. A. (2008). Nosology and diagnosis of Rett syndrome. *Research in Autism Spectrum Disorders*, 2, 601-611.

McGrew, J. H., & Keyes, M. L. (2014). Caregiver stress during the first year after diagnosis of an autism spectrum disorder. *Research in Autism Spectrum Disorders*, 8, 1373-1385.

Moss, J., & Howlin, P. (2009). Autism spectrum disorders in genetic syndromes: Implications for diagnosis, intervention and understanding the wider autism spectrum disorder population. *Journal of Intellectual Disability Research*, 53, 852-873.

Muhle, R., Trentacoste, S. V., & Rapin, I. (2004). The genetics of autism. *Pediatrics*, 113, 472-486.

Mulroy, S., Robertson, L., Aiberti, K., Leonard, H., & Bower, C. (2008). The impact of having a sibling with an intellectual disability: Parental perspectives in two disorders. *Journal of Intellectual Disability Research*, 52, 216-229.

Neul, J. L., Kaufmann, W. E., Glaze, D. G., Christodoulou, J., Clarke, A. J., Bahi-Buisson,N., et al. (2010). Rett syndrome: Revised diagnostic criteria and nomenclature. *Annals of Neurology*, 68, 944–949.

Nissenkorn, A., & Ben-Zeev, B. (2013). Unilateral rhythmic hand tapping in Rett syndrome: Is this stereotypy? *Journal of Child Neurology*, 28, 1210-1214.

Quest, K. M., Byiers, B. J., Payen, A., & Symons, F. J. (2014). *Rett syndrome: A preliminary analysis of stereotypy, stress, and negative affect. Research in Developmental Disabilities*, 35, 1191-1197.

Reichle, J. (2011). Evaluating assistive technology in the education of persons with severe disabilities. *Journal of Behavioral Education*, 20, 77-85.

Rett., A. (1966). U¨ber ein eigenartiges hirnatrophisches syndrom bei hyperamonaemie im kindesalter. Wiener Medizinische Wochenschrift, 116, 723–728.

Ryan, D., McGregor, F., Akermanis, M., Southwell, K., Ramke, M., & Woodyatt, G. (2004). Facilitating communication in children with multiple disabilities: Three case studies of girls with Rett syndrome. *Disability and Rehabilitation*, 26, 1268-1277.

Schaefer-Campion, C., & Johnson, N. L. (in press). Fostering ambulation for a preschool child with Rett syndrome: A case report. Physical & Occupational Therapy in Pediatrics. DOI:10.3109/01942638. 2014. 899287.

Shapiro, J. R., Bibat, G., Hiremath, G., Blue, M. E., Hundalani, S., Yablonski, T., et al. (2010). Bone mass in Rett syndrome: Association with clinical parameters and MECP2 mutations. *Pediatric Research*, 68, 446-451.

Shea, V. (2004). A perspective on the research literature related to early intensive behavioral intervention (Lovaas) for young children with autism. *Autism*, 8, 349-367.

Shetty, A. K., Chatters, R., Tilton, A. H., & Lacassie, Y. (2000). Syndrome of microcephaly, mental retardation, and tracheoesophageal fistula associated with features of Rett syndrome. *Journal of Child Neurology*, 15, 61-63.

Sigafoos, J., Green, V. A., Schlosser, R., O'Reilly, M. F., Lancioni, G. E., Rispoli, M., et al. (2009). Communication intervention in Rett syndrome: A systematic review. *Research in Autism Spectrum Disorders*, 3, 304–318.

Sigafoos, J., Kagohara, D.,Van Der Meer, L., Green, V. A., O'Reilly, M. F., Lancioni, G. E., et al. (2011). Communication assessment for individuals with Rett syndrome: A systematic review. *Research in Autism Spectrum Disorders*, 5, 692–700.

Sigafoos, J., Lancioni, G. E., O'Reilly, M. F., Achmadi, D., Stevens, M., Roche, L., et al. (2013). Teaching two boys with autism spectrum disorders to request the continuation of toy play using an iPad®-based speech-generating device. *Research in Autism Spectrum Disorders*, 7, 923-930.

Stasolla, F. Caffò, A.O., Picucci, L., Bosco A. (2013). Assistive Technology for promoting choice behaviors with three children with severe communication impairments. *Research in Developmental Disabilities*, 34, 2694-2700.

Stasolla, F., & Caffò, A. O. (2013). Promoting adaptive behaviours by two girls with Rett syndrome trough a microswitch-based program. *Research in Autism Spectrum Disorders*, 7, 1265-1272.

Stasolla, F., Damiani, R., & Caffò, A. O. (2014). Promoting constructive engagement by two boys with autism spectrum disorders and high functioning through behavioural interventions. *Research in Autism Spectrum Disorders*, 8, 376-380.

Stasolla, F., Damiani, R., Perilli, V., Di Leone, A., Albano, V., Stella, A., & Damato, C. (2014). Technological supports to promote choice opportunities by two children with fragile x syndrome and severe to profound developmental disabilities. *Research in Developmental Disabilites*, 35, 2993-3000.

Stasolla, F., De Pace, C., Damiani, R., Di Leone, A., Albano, V., & Perilli V. (2014). Comparing PECS and VOCA to promote communication opportunities and to reduce stereotyped behaviors by three girls with Rett syndrome. *Research in Autism Spectrum Disorders*, 8, 1269-1278.

Stasolla, F., Perilli, V., & Damiani, R. (2014). Self monitoring to promote on-task behaviour by two high functioning boys with autism spectrum disorders and symptoms of ADHD. *Research in Autism Spectrum Disorders*, 8, 472-479.

Stasolla, F., Perilli, V., Di Leone, A., Damiani, R., Albano, V., Stella, A., & Damato, C. (2015). Technological aids to support choice strategies by three girls with rett syndrome. *Research in Developmental Disabilities*, 36, 36-44.

Temudo, T., Oliveira, P., Santos, M., Dias, K., Vieira, J., Moreira, A., et al. (2007). Stereotypies in Rett syndrome: Analysis of 83 patients with and without detected MECP2 mutations. *Neurology*, 68, 1183-1187.

Wales, L., Charman, T., & Mount, R. H. (2004). An analogue assessment of repetitive hand behaviours in girls and young women with Rett syndrome. *Journal of Intellectual Disability Research*, 48, 672-678.

Young, D., Bebbington, A., DeKlerk, N., Bower, C., Nagarajan, L., & Leonard, H. (2011). The relationship between MECP2 mutation type and health status and service use trajectories over time in a Rett syndrome population. *Research in Autism Spectrum Disorders* ,5, 442–449.

In: Rett Syndrome and Other Communication ... ISBN: 978-1-63463-920-0
Editor: Daniel L. Kolby

Chapter 3

Microvascular Modifications in Rett Syndrome

G. Bianciardi[1*], M. Acampa[2] and M. Pastorelli[3]
[1]Dpt. Biotecnologie mediche, Anatomia Patologica,
Università di Siena, Siena, Italy
[2]Dpt. Scienze Neurologiche e Sensoriali,
Azienda Ospedaliera Universitaria Senese, Siena, Italy
[3]Dpt. Scienze mediche, chirurgiche e neuroscienze,
Università di Siena, Siena, Italy

Abstract

In 1990 Dieler R. et al., described in conjunctival, muscle and peripheral artery biopsies examined by light and electron microscopy, amorphous and membranous electron-dense deposits in capillaries of Rett syndrome (RTT) patients. Subclinical myocardial dysfunctions in RTT have been recently described in the patients, together with modification of the perfusion index. The presence of cold hands and feet, and blue, is a non-neurological phenotype that characterize RTT up to now not well explained. In order to evaluate the state of the microvascularity in RTT we have performed a complexity analysis of the microvasculature in the patients. By nailfold videocapillaroscopy we observed dilated capillaries and irregular, chaotic microvascular patterns.

* Corresponding author, Email: giorgio.bianciardi@unisi.it.

To quantify these features we have performed a nonlinear analysis of the images. Entropy resulted higher in Rett females than in sex- and age-matched healthy individuals ($p<0.001$). In RTT patients subtle modifications of the microvascular system are present, aspects that deserve to be deeply investigated.

Keywords: Rett syndrome, microvessels, entropy, fractal analysis, complexity analysis, morphometry

1. Introduction

Rett syndrome (RTT) is one of the most common forms of childhood neurodevelopmental disorder with a 300-fold increased risk of sudden death [1,2]: the evidence of cardiac autonomic nervous system (ANS) alterations [3,4] and cardiac arrhythmias [5] might be the underlying pathogenetic mechanism of these sudden death.

However, there are clinical and experimental evidences that, in RTT, ANS is abnormal at various levels: Rett children have small, cold, and/or blue or red hands and feet, facial flushing, dilated pupils during periods of agitation, abnormal sweating, gastrointestinal dysfunction, urinary retention [6].

In effect, RTT frequently presents, together with the reductions in skeletal growth, costipation and contracted joins, the midbrain and upper brainsteam hypo-perfusion and poor circulation, which lead to bluish tints to their feet and legs [7]. Hydrotherapy and physiotherapy to the extremities is often used to regain proper circulation and helps to keep their extremities limber [8].

Dieler R. *et al.*, described in conjunctival, muscle, and peripheral artery biopsies, examined by light and electron microscopy, amorphous and membranous electron-dense deposits in capillaries [9]. Recently a modification of perfusion index, attributed to altered peripheral vaso-constriction and intravascular volume status, was reported in RTT patients [10].

Interestingly, altered function of the peripheral microcirculation has been recently observed in a symptomatic MeCP2 knockout mouse model, indicating that these animals are characterized by an altered endothelium-dependent relaxation caused by a reduced Nitric Oxide availability, caused by an increased intravascular Reactive Oxygen Species (ROS) generation [11]

To further investigate on the microvascular involvement in RTT, we have performed a nailfold capillaroscopy in RTT and in healthy subjects, in order to determine the entropy of their microvascular patterns.

2. Material and Methods

Patients

In this study we included 70 females, mean age of 9.3 years (*SD* = 4.5; range 4.1 – 17.9 years), with a clinical diagnosis of typical RTT, based on revised criteria for this disorder [12], and 50 age-matched healthy females. All the subjects with any pathologies able to modify the morphologic appearance of the microvascular pattern (e.g. diabetic microangiopathy, hypertension, connective tissue diseases) were excluded.

Nailfold Capillaroscopy

Nailfold capillaroscopy was performed with a VideoCap (DS Medica, Italy), giving a total magnification of x 200. All observations were performed with the subjects in a costant temperature setting (22° to 25°C) after proper acclimatization as reported in Pasqui *et al.*, [13,14]. From the images collected, images of three fields for subject were randomly chosen and stored.

Image Analysis

Manual outline of the two-dimensional microvascular pattern's trajectories was performed using Adobe Photoshop on a 17" screen by two operators who were unaware of the subject's category. Non-readable areas were < 10% of the total area. Images were processed to threshold the vessel pattern without background interference and microvessel patterns were subsequently converted into outlines of single pixels, using JMicroVision 1.27 software (www.microvision.com) (figure 1).

Entropy (information dimension) was determined in the microvascular pattern.

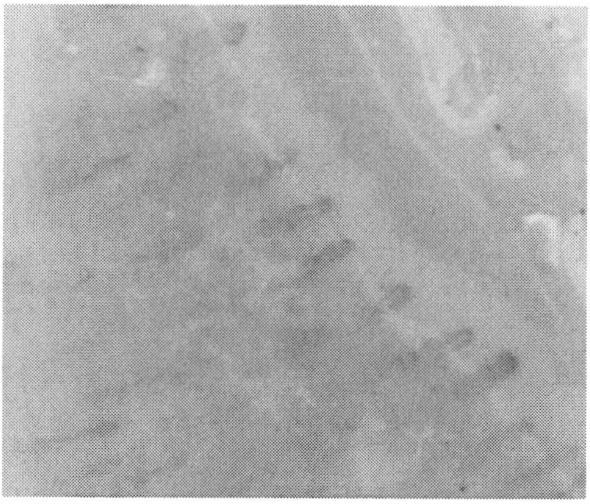

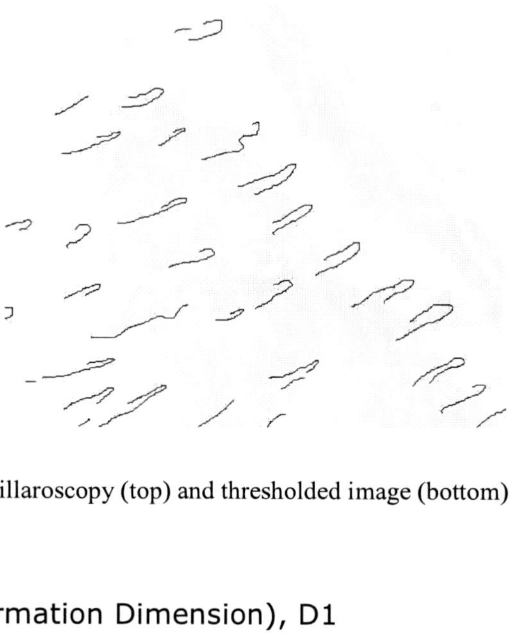

Figure 1. Videocapillaroscopy (top) and thresholded image (bottom) in a control subject (x 200).

Entropy (Information Dimension), D1

To evaluate the information (entropy) present in the patterns, information dimension, D1, a robust estimate from a finite amount of data that gives the probability of finding a point [15], was calculated using the Benoit 1.3 software (TruSoft Int'l Inc: http://trusoft-international.com/benoit.html). The box-counting algorithm was performed. To measure D1 the set is covered with boxes of linear size, d, from 9 to 100 pixels, keeping track of the mass mi (the amount of pixels) in each box, and calculates the information entropy I(d) from the summation of the number of points in the i-th box divided by the total number of points in the set multiplied for its logarithm [15, 16]. The slope of the log-log plot of information entropy vs. 1/box side length represents the information dimension of the distribution (figure 2). The method was validated by measuring computer generated Euclidean and fractal shapes of known information dimensions. Even here, a log-log straight line ($p<0.001$) revealed the statistical self-similarity of the textures.

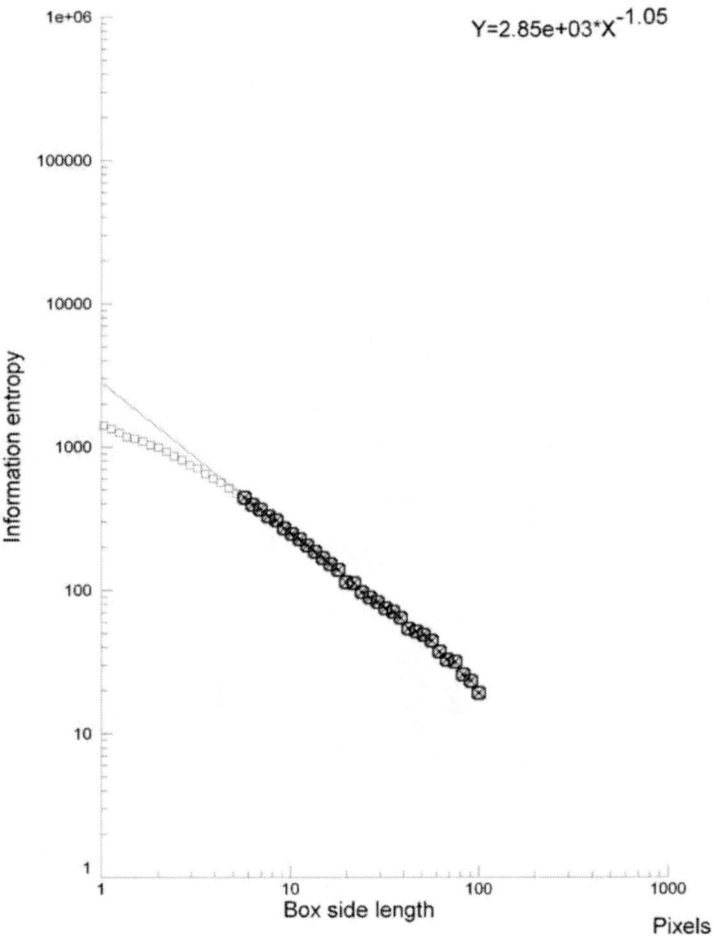

Figure 2. A log-log plot, The straight line ($p<0.001$) reveals the statistical self-similarity of the texture (the microvascular pattern is fractal), the slope is the information dimension, or entropy (Benoit 1.3 software, TruSoft Int'l Inc: http://trusoft-international.com/benoit.html). Microvascular pattern in a healthy patient (the same of Figure 1).

Statistical Analysis

Entropy indexes from the images of each subject were averaged. Mann-Whitney test was applied in order to verify significant differences between the groups. The vascular pattern analysis was reproducible, with mean intra- and inter-observer coefficient of variation of 3 % and 5 %, respectively.

3. Results

Figure #3 represents the characteristic aspect of the microvascular pattern in a Rett patient. In RTT the microvascular pattern appeared less ordered, more irregular, chaotic in appearance. Ramified and bushy capillaries were observed, some capillaries appeared giant or dilated (figure 3).

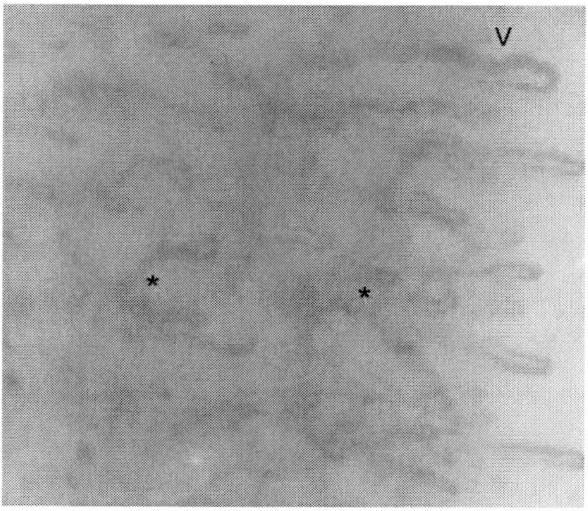

Figure 3. In RTT the microvascular pattern is often less ordered, more irregular, chaotic than in control subjects, where the pattern is ordered, with a regular distribution (compare to Figure 1). In RTT, some capillaries are giant, dilated (V) or ramified (*) in appearance. RTT patient, nailfold videocapillaroscopy, x 200.

Table #1 and figure #4 report the entropy evaluation (D1) of the microvascular pattern in healthy and Rett syndrome subjects. The studied microvascular pattern is fractal (or self-similar, see figure 2, [15]) and fractal analysis show significantly higher entropy index in Rett syndrome patients than in healthy subjects (Rett syndrome, n = 70, D1 = 1.39 (1.22 – 1.65) ; controls, n = 50, D1 = 1.16 (0.98 – 1.32); $p<0.001$).

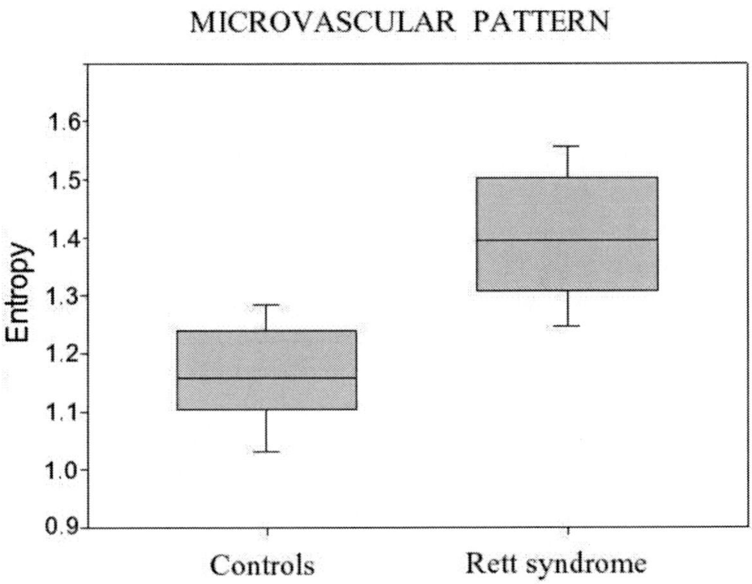

Figure 4. Box Plot, median + outliers (5th and 95th percentile). Entropy, Controls vs. Rett syndrome, $p<0.001$.

Table 1. Entropy (Information Dimension, D1, median (minimum value – maximum value) in RTT and in healthy subjects

		D1, median (min value – max value)	
Healthy subject	n = 50	1.16 (0.98 – 1.32)	
Rett syndrome	n = 70	1.39 (1.22 – 1.65)	$p < 0.001$

Information Entropy of the microvascular pattern is higher in Rett syndrome than in age-matched healthy individuals ($p<0.001$).

4. Discussion

Fractal geometry has been used for many years to perform diagnosis and prognosis, also in our hands [17-24]. In this work, a complexity index- was able to statistically distinguish Rett individuals and control ones, appearing able to assess and to quantitatively evaluate the morphological modifications of the capillaries in the RTT patients.

The findings of the present study indicate the presence of microvascular pattern abnormalities in Rett syndrome patients: often, the microvascular pattern appears chaotic and less ordered, the entropy of the microvascular pattern results higher in the patients than in age-matched normal individuals, confirming our previous results [25]. The high entropy values observed by us indicates a high complex microvascular pattern in RTT, or, in other words, the presence in the patients of a microvascular pattern more rich and less ordered in Rett individuals than in healthy age-matched controls.

Our findings may be the results of the altered peripheral vasoconstriction and hypo-perfusion described by some Authors [7,10], in an attempt to adapt in order to restore the homeostasis. We cannot also deny the importance of the autonomic nervous system that in RTT results abnormal at various levels, from the central to the peripheral nervous system [4,6]. Possible changes of the extracellular matrix (ECM) might be also be involved: we have frequently observed microvascular pattern changes in patients with extracellular matrix modifications [26-30] and a close relationship between the ECM and blood vessel network geometry has been reported [31,32].

Conclusion

It's rising the awareness that in RTT, a genetic disorder of synapse development that influence locomotor, respiratory, and cardiac functions, an impairment of microcirculation is present, as some Authors have been reported at morphological and functional levels, in patients [7,9,10] as well as in a MeCP2 null mouse model [11]. Now, our findings demonstrates that in Rett syndrome the microvascular pattern is more irregular, chaotic, less ordered, than in age-matched controls. In RTT, a cohort of subtle modifications in the microvascular system is present: an aspect that deserves to be deeply investigated.

References

[1] Acampa, M; Guideri, F. Cardiac disease and Rett syndrome. *Arch. Dis. Child*, 2006; 91, 440-443.

[2] Kerr, AM,; Stephenson, JBP. Rett's syndrome in the West of Scotland. *BMJ*, 1985; 291:579–582.

[3] Guideri, F; Acampa, M; Hayek, G; Zappella, M; Di Perri T. Reduced heart rate variability in patients affected with Rett syndrome. A possible explanation for sudden death. *Neuropediatrics* 1999; 30, 146-148.

[4] Acampa, M; Guideri, F. Autonomic nervous system alterations in Rett syndrome. *Curr. Pediatr. Rev.,* 2009; 5, 160-168.

[5] Guideri, F, Acampa, M. Sudden death and cardiac arrhythmias in Rett syndrome. *Pediatr. Cardiol.* 2005; 26, 111-119.

[6] Dahlström, A. The central and peripheral autonomic nervous system and possible implications in Rett syndrome patients. In: Kerr A, Witt-Engerström I, Eds, Rett disorder and the developing brain. Oxford University Press, Oxford: 2001; pp. 227-50.

[7] Lappalainen, R: Liewendahl, K; Sainio, K; Nikkinen, P; Riikonen, RS. Brain perfusion SPECT and EEG findings in Rett syndrome. *Acta Neurol. Scand*, 1997; 95, 44–50.

[8] Bumin, G; Uyanik, M; Yilmaz, I; Kayihan, H; Topcu, M. Hydrotherapy for Rett syndrome. *J. Rehabil Med*, 2003; 35, 44–45.

[9] Dieler, R; Schröder, JM; Reddemann, K.. Electron-dense lipidic capillary deposits in Rett syndrome. *Acta Neuropathol.*, 1990; 79, 573-578.

[10] De Felice, C; Maffei, S; C. Signorini et al., Subclinical myocardial dysfunction in Rett syndrome. *Eur. Heart J. Cardiovasc. Imaging*, 2012; 13, 339-345.

[11] Panighini, A; Duranti, E; Santini, F; Maffei, M; Pizzorusso, T et al., Vascular Dysfunction in a Mouse Model of Rett Syndrome and Effects of Curcumin Treatment. *PLoS ONE,* 2013; 8(5): e64863. doi:10.1371/journal.pone.0064863.

[12] Williamson, SL; Christodoulou, J. Rett syndrome: new clinical and molecular insights. *Eur. J. Hum. Genet*, 2006; 14, 896-903.

[13] Pasqui, AL; Puccetti, L; Di Renzo, M; Bruni, F; Camarri, A et al., Structural and functional abnormality of systemic microvessels in cardiac syndrome X. *Nutr. Metable Cardiovasc. Dis.* 2005; 15(1): 56-64.

[14] Pasqui, AL; Pastorelli, M; Puccetti, L; Beerman, U; Biagi, F et al., Microvascular assessment in Behçet disease: videocapillaroscopic study. *Int. J. Tissue React.* 2003;25(3):105-115.
[15] Falconer, K. Fractal geometry: Mathematical Foundations and Applications. Chichester, John Wiley, 1990.
[16] Pitsianis, N; Bleris, GL; Argyrakis, P. Information dimension in fractal structures. *Phys. Rev. B*, 1989; 39 (10), 7097-7100.
[17] Cross, SS; Cotton, DWK. The fractal dimension may be a useful morphometric discriminant in histopathology. *J. Path*, 1992; 166, 409-411.
[18] Cross, SS; Bury, JP; Silcocks, PB; Stephenson, TJ; Cotton, DWK. Fractal geometric analysis of colorectal polyps. *J. Path*, 1994; 172, 317-323.
[19] Losa, GA., Nonnenmacher, TF. Self-similarity and fractal irregularity in pathologic tissues. *Mod. Pathol*, 1996; 9, 174 - 182.
[20] Bianciardi, G: Miracco, C; De Santi, MM; Luzi, P. Differential diagnosis between mycosis fungoides and chronic dermatitis by fractal analysis. *J. Dermatol. Sci.*, 2003; 33, 184–86.
[21] Bianciardi, G; Tanganelli, I; Totagiancaspro, D; Brogi, M et al., Fractal analysis of monocytes in diabetes. *Clin. Hemorheol. Microcirc.* 35 (2006), 269 – 272.
[22] Bianciardi, G; Bisogno, S; Bertoldi, I; Laurini, L; Coviello, G; Frediani, B. Fractal dimension of bone texture in radiographs correlates to ultrasound broadband attenuation T-score. *Clin. Exp. Rheumatol.*, 2013; 31, 389-393.
[23] Bianciardi, G; Miracco, C; Lazzi, S; Luzi, P. Fractal analysis of epithelial-connective tissue interface in basal cell carcinoma of the skin. *Curr. Bioinformatics*, 2013; 8, 357-361.
[24] Bianciardi, G; Luzi, P. Fractal analysis of the bone marrow in myelodysplastic syndromes. *Curr. Bioinformatics*, 2014; 9(4), 408-413.
[25] Bianciardi G; Acampa, M; Lamberti, I; Sartini, S et al., Microvascular abnormalities in Rett syndrome. *Clin. Hemor Microcirc.*, 2013; 54, 109-113.
[26] De Felice, C; Latini, G; Bianciardi, G et al., Abnormal vascular network complexity: A new phenotypical marker in hereditary nonpolyposis colorectal cancer syndrome. *Gut*, 2003; 52, 1764 – 1767.
[27] De Felice, C; Bianciardi, G; Laurini, R; Parrini, S; Latini, G. Congenital oral mucosal abnormalities in newborns with true umbilical cord knots. *Biol. Neonate*, 2004; 86, 34 – 38.

[28] De Felice, C; Parrini, S; Di Maggio, G; Bianciardi, G et al., Oral mucosal microvascular network abnormalities in de novo mutation achondroplasia. *Fractals*, 2005; 13, 73 – 82.
[29] Latini, G; Bianciardi, G; Parrini, S et al., Abnormal oral vascular network pattern geometry: a new clinical sign of Down Syndrome. *J. Pediatr,* 2006; 148, 132–137.
[30] Bianciardi, G; Traversi, C; Cattaneo, R; De Felice, C et al., Phase transition of Microvascular Network Architecture in Human Pathologies. *Theor. Biol. Forum*, 2012: 1, 37 – 45.
[31] Ingber, DE; Folkman, J. Mechanochemical switching between growth and differentiation during fibroblast growth factor-stimulated angiogenesis *in vitro*: Role of extracellular matrix. *J. Cell Biol.*, 1984; 109, 317–330.
[32] Suwa, N. Supracellular structural principle and geometry of blood vessels. *Virchows Arch. A,* 1981; 390, 161–179.

Index

D

E

F

G

H

I

J

K

L

Q

R

S

T

U

V

W

X

Y